# Pregnant And Lovin' It

by
Lindsay R. Curtis, M.D.
and
Yvonne Coroles, R.N.
Illustrated by
Paul Farber

W9-CNZ-149

Published by H.P. Books, P.O. Box 5367, Tucson, Arizona 85703 USA
ISBN: 0-912656-82-4 H.P. Book Number 82, Library of Congress Catalog Card
Number: 77-82-12 © 1977 by Lindsay R. Curtis. Printed in U.S.A. 7-77

# Preface

You are about to embark upon the greatest—and hopefully—the most pleasurable experience of your entire life. Giving birth to a baby can be the most exciting and also the most rewarding event in a woman's life.

Most of the joy of having a baby is the anticipation, but this can only be so if a mother is free of fear and full of confidence. This book is written to answer the commonest questions that arise in pregnancy. It is not intended to be encyclopedic.

But if it can answer enough of your questions to set your mind at ease, its purpose will have been accomplished.

# Introduction

If you want to know the questions that trouble pregnant women... ask a woman who is pregnant. Through our Childbirth Education Classes each year pass about 2000 women... and their husbands. In each of the eight lectures and demonstrations they are encouraged to ask questions.

This book, in question and answer form, is the result of sifting, sorting, and selecting through the many questions asked each year. We think you will find the answer to your question among them.

In cooperation with the authors, artist Paul Farber has carried the petite star of our book along with her pet poodle through many of the trials, triumphs and emoluments of pregnancy. We hope you will find it first of all informative... but also entertaining.

# 1 | *It Has To Start Somewhere!*

### 1. *How Soon Should I Go To The Doctor?*

Some doctors prefer to see you after you have missed two menstrual periods. It is difficult to tell for sure about pregnancy if you are examined too soon after missing your first menstrual period.

However, most women become very anxious and nervous if they go two weeks over their period. If you are terribly anxious about your condition, phone your doctor and he will see you sooner.

### 2. *How Early Will The Pregnancy Test Be Positive?*

It usually will not be positive until about 10 days after you have missed your first menstrual period. Nor is the pregnancy test 100% accurate. About 95% to 98% accuracy is average.

A pregnancy test is not performed routinely unless there is some compelling reason. The doctor can ordinarily rely upon his clinical findings to determine if you are pregnant.

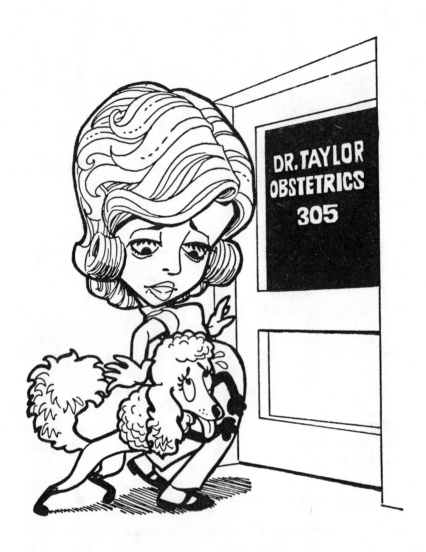

*How Soon Should I Go To The Doctor?*

### 3.   Other Than Missing A Menstrual Period, What Are Other Early Signs of Pregnancy?

Don't rely completely on a missed menstrual period, since this is not always dependable, either way. In addition to missing a menstrual period you may notice:

a. Morning sickness

b. Engorgement and soreness of your breasts

c. Easy fatigue

d. Frequent urination (you may also have to get up in the middle of the night to urinate)

e. Dark discoloration of the skin in the disc around your nipples.

f. Anxiety is common, but varies with the individual

Admittedly these signs and symptoms vary with each expectant mother and other symptoms may be observed as the pregnancy progresses.

### 4.   I Have Never Had A Pelvic Examination. What Should I Expect?

Remember that the pelvic examination is only one part of a complete physical examination. Your doctor will examine your head, neck, chest (including heart, lungs, and breasts), abdomen, and your arms and legs in a general way.

In a pelvic examination it is necessary that you be positioned on a special examining table, lying on your back, with your knees drawn up and your feet in stirrups (as shown in illustration). This enables your doctor to conveniently check your female organs. It helps to take a deep breath, then slowly let it out for ten counts. This will help you to relax.

After he inserts an instrument called a speculum, into the vagina, the doctor can look at the cervix (mouth of the uterus), take a cancer smear, and also tell if the cervix has undergone the typical changes of pregnancy. In pregnancy the cervix changes color from pink to blue

**3**

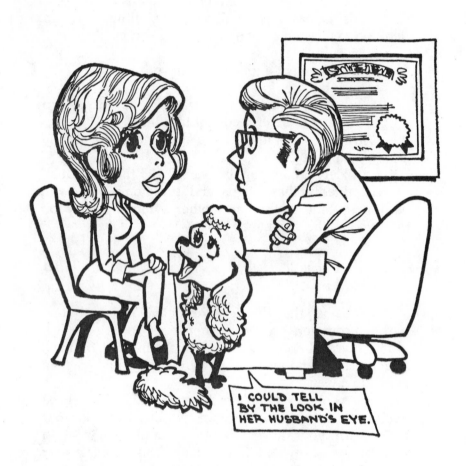

*How Early Will The Pregnancy Test Be Positive?*

and becomes softer (like the difference in the consistency between your nose and your lips).

With two fingers in the vagina and his other hand placed gently on the abdomen, he makes his pelvic examination. If you take a deep breath it will help you relax and make it easier for your doctor to better outline your uterus, tubes, and ovaries. If your abdomen is relaxed the doctor can better detect the softening changes of pregnancy in these tissues, as well as any abnormalities, such as cysts or tumors of these organs.

On certain occasions your doctor may wish to confirm the diagnosis of pregnancy with a pregnancy urine test. Such a test can be performed in his office on a "while-you-wait" basis in a matter of minutes.

**5.** *I Have A Friend Who Had All The Symptoms Of Pregnancy Yet It Was Finally Discovered That She Was Not Pregnant. How Is This Possible?*

This is called "false pregnancy" and is often found in those who greatly desire pregnancy but cannot conceive. It may also be found sometimes in those who fear pregnancy. Nature and mind play some cruel tricks on such an individual.

False pregnancy may cause vomiting, missed menstrual periods, weight gain and even quickening ("feel life"). Unfortunately these individuals must eventually face the fact that they are not pregnant.

Normal people under some circumstances experience the same sensations and symptoms. We simply have no explanation for many of these cases.

**6.** *I Have Always Wondered Where And How Fertilization Of The Egg Takes Place.*

As you know, sperm from the male are deposited in the vagina by intercourse. From this point the sperm

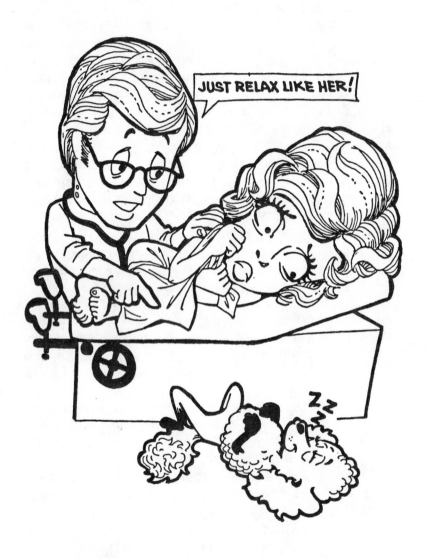

*I Have Never Had A Pelvic Examination. What Should I Expect?*

swim by means of their tail through the secretions of the vagina, making their way into the cervix.

Swimming through the secretions found on the lining of the uterus, the sperm make their way into the fallopian tube. It is in the outer part of the fallopian tube, the part farthest from the uterus, that the sperm meets the egg. Although several sperm may find their way into the tube, only one sperm penetrates the egg to effect fertilization.

From this point the now-fertilized egg makes it's way down the tube (it takes about 3 days) into the cavity of the uterus. In the meantime the fertilized egg has already divided several times and becomes a round ball of cells.

It is here in the rich and nutritious lining of the uterine cavity that the fertilized egg (after 4 or 5 days in the uterine cavity) becomes imbedded. It now begins to develop into what is called an embryo (up to 2 months), then into a fetus, and finally into a full term, fully developed baby, ready for birth.

### 7. How Long Does A Sperm Remain Alive After It Has Been Deposited In The Vagina?

Although we are not absolutely sure, it is thought that a sperm is capable of fertilization for one to two days. Sperm may remain active but immobile for longer than this.

Sperm require a lower-than-normal body temperature in which to survive. This is perhaps the reason that the testicles are on the outside of the male body.

### 8. How Long Does The Ovum (Egg) Remain Alive After It Is Released From The Ovary?

Here again we *think* it remains alive for about 24 hours, after which it dies and is discarded. Fertilization often takes place within 12 hours of ovulation.

7

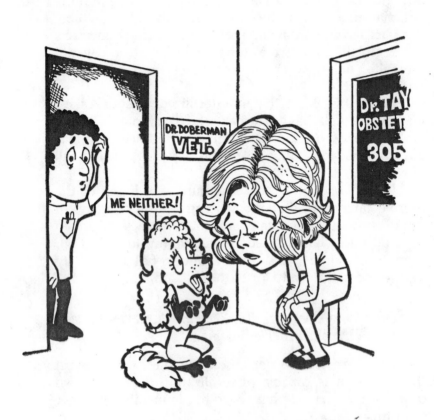

*I Have A Friend Who Had All The Symptoms Of Pregnancy Yet It Was Finally Discovered That She Was Not Pregnant. How Is This Possible?*

Some think the fertile period in the female (the time during which she could conceive) is less than 12 hours. However, there are additional factors which may influence fertility. Coitus, itself, may stimulate ovulation.

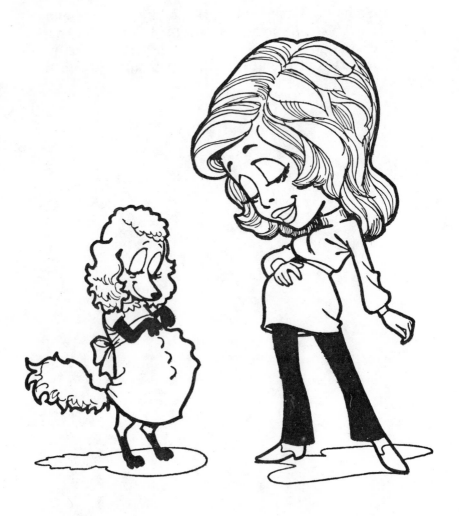

*Why Are My Breasts So Tender?*

# 2 | *What's To Become Of Me Now?*

Almost from the moment of conception a woman begins to change—physically and emotionally. Yet these changes vary with each individual woman. Let's discuss a few of them.

### 1. *Why Are My Breasts So Tender?*

One of the first signs of pregnancy is tenderness of the breasts. They feel full, become larger and more tender. This is because nature, by means of hormones, is preparing the breasts for breast feeding.

Whether you are going to breast-feed or not, your breasts are preparing for nursing just the same. Much engorgement of the breast is caused by the greater flow of blood, as well as an increased number and size of glands in the pregnant breast.

### 2. *Is It Normal To Have Secretion From My Nipples During Pregnancy?*

Yes! This is a milky secretion similar to "colostrum"

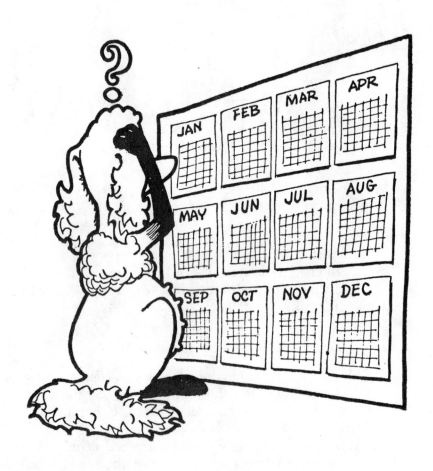

*Why Do Birth Control Pills, Taken Prior To Pregnancy, "Foul Up" Due Dates?*

a watery fluid which is the forerunner of "regular" milk produced a few days after the baby is born. It is good for the baby, although it may be a nuisance to the mother.

It can usually be controlled by inserting paper tissues in the bra to absorb this fluid. If fluid is excessive in amount, a tiny plastic dish-cover filled with paper tissue can be worn inside the bra to prevent soiling of clothing.

### 3. Why Do Birth Control Pills, Taken Prior To Pregnancy, "Foul Up" Due Dates?

It is not uncommon for a woman to miss one or several menstrual periods when she discontinues taking the birth control pill. For instance, she usually will have a menstrual period within a couple of days after discontinuing the pill, but then fail to have another one for several months.

Many of these cycles are anovulatory; in other words, no egg is released from the ovary. When ovulation resumes, a woman again becomes fertile and may become pregnant. After ovulating she then resumes her menstrual periods unless of course she has become pregnant. In such an instance, however, it may be difficult for her to know exactly from which date to calculate when her baby is due to be born.

### 4. Is There Any Way To Estimate How Large My Baby Might Be At A Given Time In My Pregnancy?

Doctors use several methods that involve centimeters and lunar months, but these are cumbersome for most people. However, here a few simple rules to follow:

One month—Half the size of the end of your little finger.

Two months—As large as the end of your thumb.

Three months—The size of your entire thumb.

13

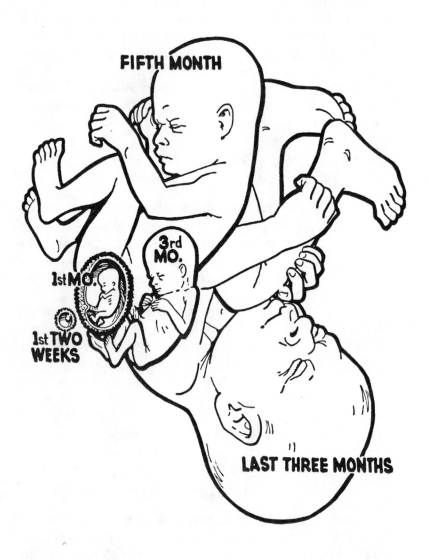

*Development of the Embryo: 0 To 8 weeks—after 8 weeks it is called a fetus.*

Four months—About the size of a frankfurter.

Five months—may weigh a little less than a pound, and is 10 inches in length.

Six months—Weighs about 1½ pounds, and is a little over one foot long.

Seven months—Weighs 2¼ pounds and is 15 inches long.

Eight months—Weighs 4-5 pounds and is 16-17 inches long.

Nine months—Weighs 6 pounds and is 19 inches long.

Ten months—Weighs 7 pounds and is 21 inches long. (Ten lunar months equal 280 days or full term)

5.  *Fertilization Of The Egg. See page 16*


6.  *Development of the Embryo: 0 To 8 weeks—after 8 weeks it is called a fetus. See page 18*


7.  *Relative Development At Various Stages Of Pregnancy. See page 18*


8.  *What Does The Doctor Mean By Trimester?*

Since the average pregnancy is about nine months in duration, this time is divided into three sections of three months each, called the first, second, and third (or last) trimester of pregnancy.

Another way of calibrating the duration of pregnancy is by lunar months, consisting of 28 days each In this case, there are ten lunar months of pregnancy, that is 28 days × 10 months = 280 days.

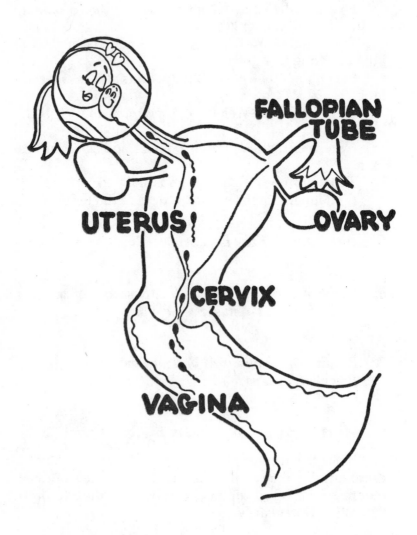

*I Have Always Wondered Where And How Fertilization Of The Egg Takes Place.*

16

### 9. What Role Does The Afterbirth Play In The Development Of The Fetus?

During its 3-day journey down the tube to the uterine cavity, the fertilized egg divides again and again. During the 3 or 4 days it remains in the cavity of the uterus, it continues to develop. By this time it has reached a stage where it requires more nourishment than the uterine secretions along the way can provide.

In the meantime it has developed some specialized cells on one side of the embryo which enable it to burrow into the wall of the uterus. Here it establishes communication with the bloodstream of the mother and the specialized cells develop into what is called the afterbirth, also known as the placenta.

The baby's blood and the mother's blood never come in direct contact with each other, but an exchange of oxygen and nourishment takes place between them through several layers of membranes in the placenta. The placenta serves as the middleman, or marketplace for this exchange.

### 10. Where Does The Bag Of Water Come In?

This is called the amniotic sac and the fluid it contains is called "amniotic fluid". The amniotic cavity starts as a tiny sac of water, but eventually this bag of water completely surrounds the baby, like pushing a fist into a soft balloon, providing a watery cushion against any temperature change, injury, pressure, or inflammation as the baby increases in size. The water also keeps the baby from rubbing against the walls of the uterus.

### 11. Where Does The Water Come From?

At first the amniotic fluid comes from the mother's blood serum but later on it receives urine from the fetus.

**17**

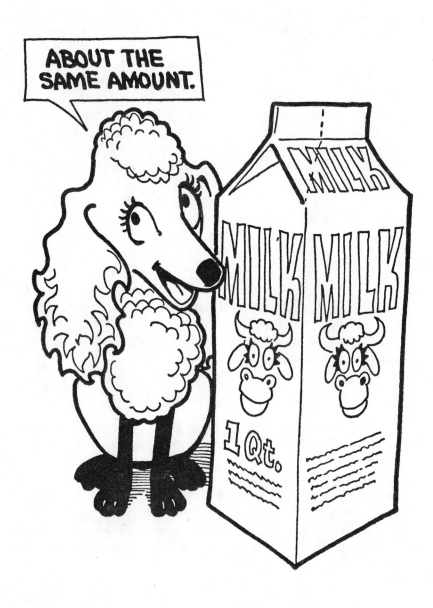

*The Average Amount Of Water In The Amniotic Sac Is A Little Over A Quart*

As the baby swallows amniotic fluid, its kidneys secrete urine into the amniotic fluid, and the process continues as the fluid is "recycled" through the kidneys.

### 12. Why Do Some Women Have More Water Than Others?

The average amount of water in the amniotic sac is a little over one quart. When this amount exceeds two quarts it is not only abnormal but it becomes somewhat uncomfortable for the mother.

Women may have only a tiny amount of water or a large amount. We don't know the reason.

### 13. Is It Dangerous To Have An Excessive Amount Of Water?

There are certain complications with excessive water. For instance, there are known to be more defective babies when there is more than the normal amount of amniotic fluid.

Also, when there is excessive water, there is greater likelihood that the bag of water will break with a gush even before labor begins. At this time the umbilical cord may "wash" past the baby and into the vagina. With subsequent labor contractions, the blood vessels in the cord then become compressed between the baby's head (or breech) and the cervix or pelvic wall.

Unless this compression is relieved and blood allowed to flow through the umbilical cord, the baby will suffocate. Sometimes the baby can be saved only by immediate delivery which may require Cesarean operation.

### 14. What Is The Purpose Of The Umbilical Cord?

The cord contains blood vessels (two arteries and one vein which connect the placenta and the baby)

19

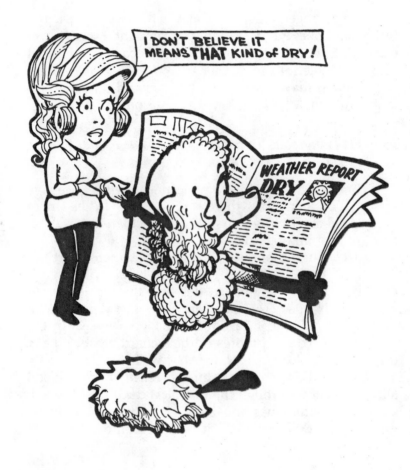

*What Is A Dry Birth And How Dangerous Is It?*

surrounded by a jellylike material. The covering of the cord is simply a continuation of the amniotic sac.

The cord varies in length from a few inches to several feet, and is about the thickness of an adult finger. The cord is the baby's lifeline, supplying it with nourishment and oxygen.

### 15. What Is A Dry Birth And How Dangerous Is It?

A true "dry" birth is almost non-existent because amniotic fluid is secreted continuously, mostly by the baby's kidneys. It is not uncommon, after the bag of water breaks, to have a great gush of amniotic fluid.

One purpose of this fluid is to "lubricate" the birth canal for passage of the baby. Because this fluid continues to be formed there is no such thing as a "dry birth".

### 16. I Have Heard That Doctors Count The Number Of Blood Vessels In The Umbilical Cord. Why Is This Important?

Normally, there are two arteries (carrying blood from the baby to the placenta). About one baby in 100 has only one artery in the cord.

But of the babies who have only one artery, 25% have birth defects. For this reason, doctors always check to see if all three blood vessels (two arteries and one vein) are present in the cord.

### 17. What Is A Prolapsed Cord?

This is a condition in which the umbilical cord becomes compressed between the presenting part of the baby (usually the head), and the wall of the pelvis, thus shutting off the blood supply to the baby. Such a condition requires immediate delivery of the baby, either vaginally or by Cesarean operation.

21

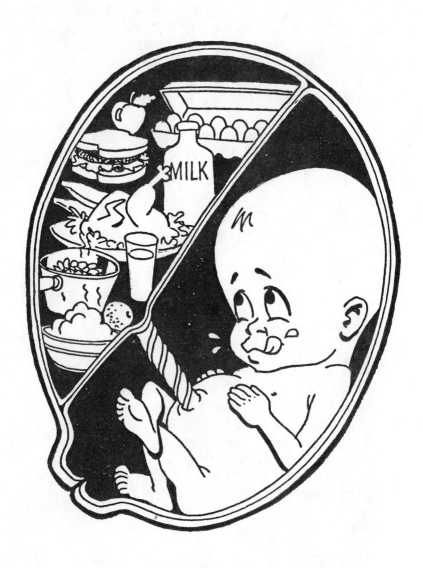

*If the Baby Is Encased In Water How Does It Get Food And How Does It Eliminate Waste?*

## 18. If The Baby Is Encased In Water How Does It Get Food And How Does It Eliminate Waste?

Its nourishment comes completely from the mother through the placenta and into the baby's blood supply through the umbilical cord. Oxygen likewise is carried by the blood through the cord.

Waste in a fetus is minimal and is accumulated in the baby's bowel as a tarry, greenish-black material, called meconium. Normally it is not eliminated from the bowel as a stool until birth, unless the baby is subjected to stress or strain. Most often such stress occurs if the cord is compressed, causing the baby to struggle in its futile attempt to breathe.

Urine from the fetus is eliminated into the amniotic fluid surrounding the baby.

## 19. What Are The Soft Spots In The Baby's Head?

These are called "fontanels" and mark the juncture of the various bones of the baby's head. The bones of the head are purposely "un-joined" before birth so that they can "give" during delivery. These bones may even overlap each other, if necessary, as the baby's head is compressed in order to pass through the birth canal.

The soft spots have no particular significance except that if the baby becomes markedly dehydrated, these tend to withdraw somewhat. The size of the soft spots is not too important.

Generally these fontanels close spontaneously as the bones grow together and cover these spaces. Most often this process is complete by about 18 months of age.

## 20. How Fast Does The Fetus Grow And Develop?

First two weeks: the egg is dividing rapidly and soon becomes a ball of cells (has a large yolk sac for nutrition). This sphere of cells quickly develops an amniotic sac that

23

presently envelops what is now called the embryo. At this stage the embryo and sac have a relationship similar to a fist pushed into a small balloon containing water. The part of the balloon over the fist develops into skin covering the fetus and the rest of the balloon becomes the amniotic sac.

Third week: Heart, brain, and rudimentary limbs develop. Rudimentary tail is still present.

Fourth week: Rapid growth with development of first traces of eyes, ears, nose and all other organs.

Second month (4 to 8 weeks): marked growth of head size in proportion to body. Heart begins to beat and circulation begins.

Third month (8 to 12 weeks): Fingers and toes are recognizable with soft nails. Movements of fetus begin. Sex organs begin to develop, but sex cannot be determined except by microscope.

Fourth month (12 to 16 weeks):
    1—Sex is recognizable by now.
    2—Fetus is 4 to 6 inches in length.
    3—Vagina and anus are patent (open).
    4—Some digestion begins.

Fifth month (16 to 20 weeks):
    1—Downy covering of hair over body with slightly more on top of head.
    2—The eyelids are still fused.

Sixth month (20 to 24 weeks):
    1—Thin, reddish, wrinkled skin with beginning fat deposit under it.
    2—Head is still large compared with the body.
    3—If born, baby will attempt to breathe, but will not survive.

Seventh month (24 to 28 weeks):
    1—Skin is covered with "cheesy" material, called vernix.
    2—Covering membrane disappears from eyes.
    3—Eyelids separated.
    4—Sight and hearing are usually the last things

24

to develop, but should be all right now.

5—If born, baby occasionally survives.

Eighth month (28 to 32 weeks):

1—Skin still looks like "little old man" because of lack of fat under it.

2—Baby is likely to survive with good care; however, at this stage, the baby is still subject to atelectasis, a condition in which the lung is not mature enough to expand as it should.

Ninth month (32-36 weeks):

1—Face no longer wrinkled.

2—If born now, it should survive.

Tenth month (36 to 40 weeks):

1—Skin is smooth, has lost most of the down except over shoulders.

2—Hair likely to be dark.

3—Covered with vernix (cheesy material).

4—Nails have grown beyond finger and toe tips.

5—Testicles are in scrotum in male. Lips of vagina are developed and touch each other in the female.

6—Skull bones are calcified.

7—Eyes are slate-colored. Impossible to predict ultimate color.

## 21. Do Boys Really Weigh More At Birth Than Girls?

Yes. Average is about 3 ounces more.

## 22. Can Sex Be Determined Before Birth?

Yes. By withdrawing some amniotic fluid through a special needle and examining it under a microscope, the sex can be determined. However, this is done only for medical reasons where a sex-linked defect, such as hemophilia, is involved. Surveys show that couples

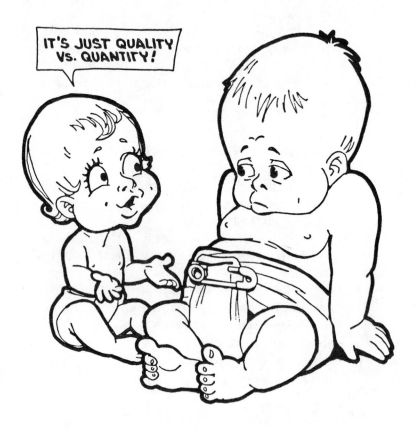

*Do Boys Really Weigh More At Birth Than Girls?*

would not like to know the sex of their baby before birth. (They still like the "guessing" game).

### 23. Can Sex Be Pre-Determined? In Other Words, Can We Plan Conception So We Will Have One Or The Other?

There is some evidence now to indicate that coitus at the exact time of ovulation (14 days before the onset of the next menstrual period) is more likely to produce a male infant. Coitus before this time is more likely to produce a girl. An alkaline pre-coital douche seems to be more favorable for production of a male, and an acid douche for the female.

### 24. Does A Baby Breathe Before It Is Born—(While It Is Being Carried By The Mother)?

Yes. It does not breathe air, of course. However, rhythmic respiratory movements may occur as early as 12 weeks and continue until birth. After it is born, the baby simply continues doing what it has already been doing, but with considerably more effort, as it breathes air.

### 25. Do All Babies Have Hiccups?

Babies do have hiccups frequently before birth. It is a common reflex effect on the diaphragm. Some babies are more prone to this than others.

### 26. Does The Baby Produce Urine Before It Is Born?

Yes. And this is secreted into the amniotic fluid.

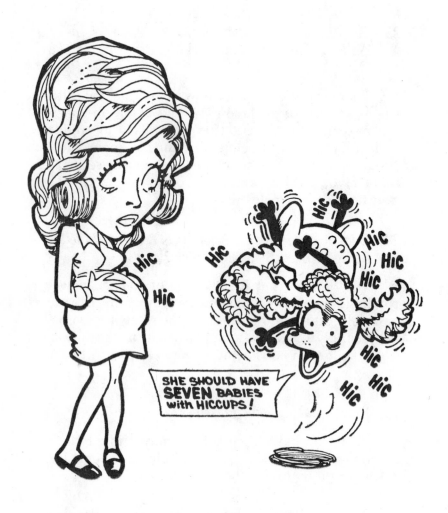

*Do All Babies Have Hiccups?*

### 27. Does The Baby Have Normal Digestion Before Birth?

Yes, to a limited extent. However, it does not have bowel movements until after birth unless asphyxia occurs causing it to struggle or strain. The fecal material produced before birth is called meconium and is retained in the intestinal tract. It looks almost like soft, black tar.

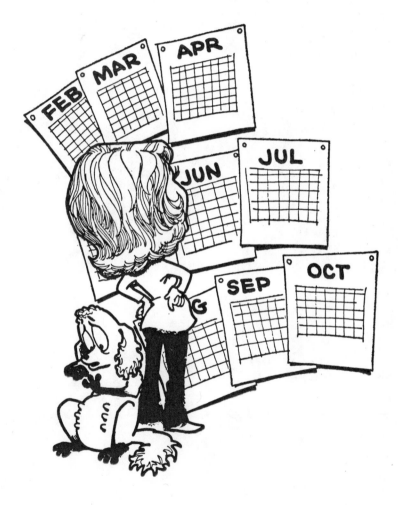

*How Far Along Am I?*

# 3 | Pregnancy Is Three Times Three

## 1. How Far Along Am I?

Pregnancy takes 280 days counting from the first day of the last menstrual period. This assumes a 28-day menstrual cycle in which ovulation (and fertilization) occur on the 14th day counting from the first day of flow. Therefore, the actual pregnancy lasts for (280 minus 14) about 266 days.

A doctor usually counts from the first day of the last menstrual period, even though the pregnancy did not begin until two weeks later. Therefore, if he says you are eight weeks pregnant, he means eight weeks from your last menstrual period, even though the embryo is only six weeks old.

Women tend to say, "I am in my fourth month," which is rather vague. It would be more accurate to say, 'I am twelve weeks (or sixteen weeks) along," which assumes she is counting from the first day of her last menstrual period.

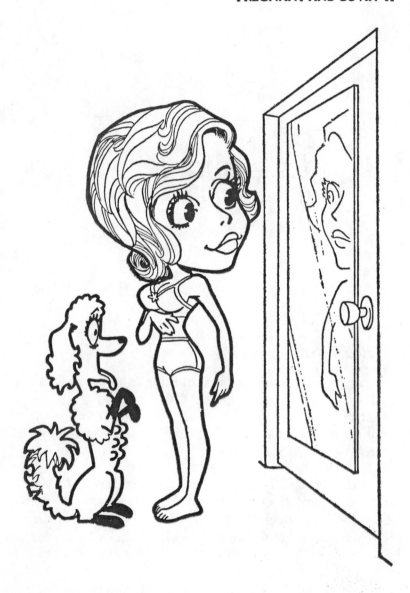

*Is There Any Way To Keep My Breasts Full Like This After My Baby?*

## 2. When Am I Due To Have My Baby?

To calculate when your baby is due to be born, most doctors count back three months from the first day of your last menstrual period and add seven days. For instance: last menstrual period began May 2nd, baby due February 9th.

It is neither uncommon nor abnormal, however, to have your baby as much as two weeks early or two weeks late. Only one woman in ten delivers on the exact "due" date.

## 3. What Are The Small Bumps Around My Nipples?

These are small glands (in the disc around the nipple) that enlarge in pregnancy. They lubricate the area around the nipple, allowing for easier, less painful nursing.

The appearance of these tubercles, as they are called, along with pigmentation of the disc surrounding the nipple are early signs of pregnancy.

## 4. What Makes Veins Of My Breasts Show Up So Much? Will These Unsightly Things Remain Permanently?

Due to engorgement of blood in the breast during pregnancy, the veins tend to show up more—especially when the superficial layer of the skin is stretched and is extra thin. When the pregnancy is over and nursing is discontinued, these veins usually disappear.

## 5. Is There Any Way To Keep My Breasts Full Like This After My Baby?

Unfortunately not. Many small-busted women have expressed this wish, but the enlargement is due to temporary engorgement.

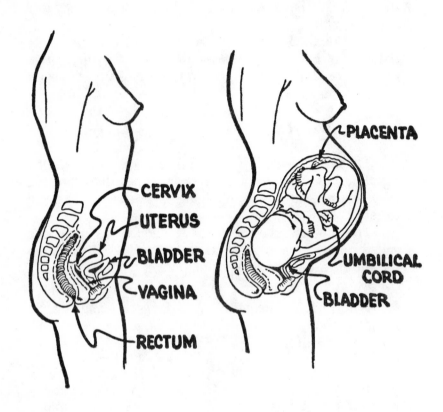

*Pressure From The Uterus On The Bladder Causes Me To Urinate So Often.*

However, with a good supportive bra, good posture, and daily breast exercises you may maintain or build even more desirable breasts.

## 6. Why Do I Have To Urinate So Often?

There is a hormonal change early in pregnancy that seems to cause frequency and urgency of urination. Later, beginning at about two months, the uterus exerts pressure on the bladder much like pressing a fist into a small, soft balloon. This pressure decreases the capacity of the bladder and gives a woman the urge to empty it, although it may contain only a small amount of urine.

This condition is relieved somewhat at about four months, as the uterus rises into the abdomen. Unfortunately the feeling returns as the baby descends into the pelvis during the last few weeks of pregnancy, again due to pressure on the bladder.

Avoid drinking fluids after four o'clock in the afternoon so that you will not be up all night. If possible drink most of your liquids in the forenoon.

## 7. Why Do I Feel So Bloated During Pregnancy And Have So Much Gas?

Smooth muscle tissue, wherever it is found, loses much of its tone during pregnancy. As a result, the muscles in the walls of the intestines become lazy and flabby.

Digestion is slowed, causing you to feel uncomfortably full, bloated and gassy. If this sensation becomes too annoying, your doctor can give you something for relief.

Deep abdominal breathing sometimes helps to move the gas. Good posture habits also help—especially try to avoid "slumping".

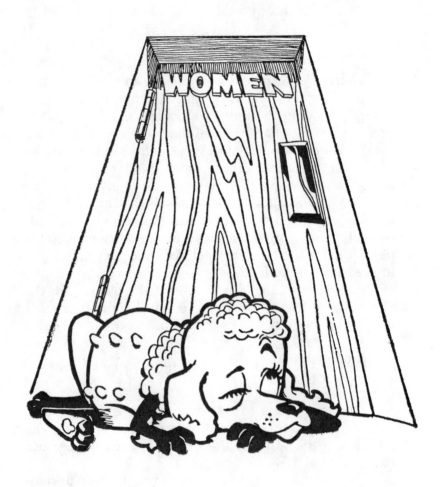

*Why Do I Have To Urinate So Often?*

**8** *Why Do I Have Heartburn? Does This Have Anything To Do With My Heart?*

Heartburn, or indigestion, has nothing to do with your heart. It is often due to the slowed digestive action of food in your stomach and upper intestines, which also encourages "gas". You may be aware of a sense of fullness or even a "burning feeling" in your throat.

A tablespoon of cream one half hour before meals sometimes relieves this discomfort. If you feel you need additional relief, a teaspoon of milk of magnesia or other antacids after meals will often help.

**9.** *Why Am I Constipated During Pregnancy When I Never Did Have This Problem Before?*

Your entire intestine functions less efficiently than it did when you were not pregnant. Since your bowel is part of the intestinal tract, it likewise fails to function as it should. Try the following suggestions:

1. Increase your fluid intake (especially fruit juices).
2. Try to develop regular bowel habits.
3. Take only the laxatives your doctor prescribes for you.
4. Bulk-forming and stool-softening laxatives may be preferable to the more irritating laxatives.
5. One tablespoon of honey in one half glass of warm water taken morning and night seems to help certain individuals.
6. Place feet up on a small stool while evacuating the the bowel. Sitting up straight is less comfortable and often less effective.

**10.** *Why Do I Cry So Easily And Become Upset And Angry Over Nothing?*

Due to hormone changes, pregnant women often become moody, depressed and easily upset. Under old

**37**

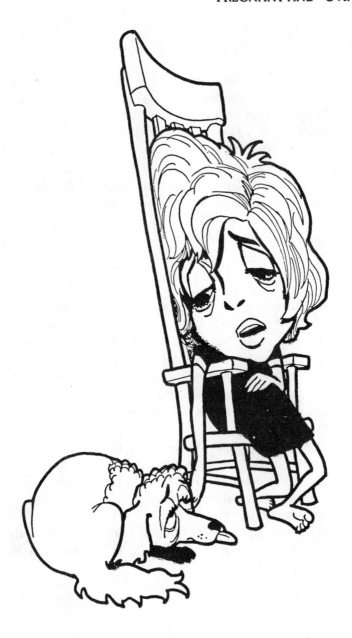

*Why Do I Tire So Easily And Require More Sleep Than Usual?*

English law, a pregnant woman's testimony was not accepted in court because she was not held to be reliable. Naturally this entire idea is exaggerated, but it does show that the emotional change in pregnant women is not something new.

Most women have a period of adjustment to make when they discover they are pregnant. Every woman does not become pregnant the exact moment she wants to. And, even if you had tried for years to have a baby, now that you are finally pregnant, you may wonder if you did the right thing.

However, be assured that you are not alone. Many women find their emotions are much more brittle during pregnancy. If you can be patient, it is comforting to know that you will return to normal with full control over your emotions after your pregnancy is over.

## 11. Why Do I Tire So Easily And Require More Sleep Than Usual?

This may be due, in part, to a loss of muscle tone throughout the body. This same fatigue is common in women who take birth control pills, perhaps because the pills simulate pregnancy.

Sometimes this is nature's way of slowing you down. With a "super-drama" like pregnancy going on in your body, you cannot always continue the fast pace you set when you were not pregnant.

However, the fatigue is a temporary condition and may be expected to disappear once the pregnancy is over. In the meantime get all the rest and exercise you can.

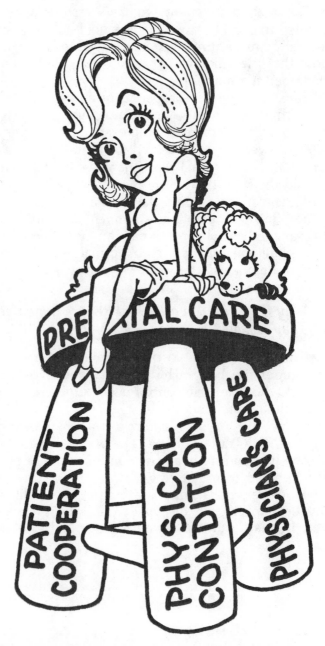

*Good Prenatal Care Is Like A Three-Legged Stool...*

# 4 | *Prenatal Care (I'm On My Way)*

Good prenatal care is like a three-legged stool, supported by (1) your physician's care, (2) your cooperation and (3) your physical condition. Hopefully all three cooperate to make it an enjoyable pregnancy.

We have already discussed your first pelvic examination. In addition to this your doctor will check your heart, lungs, breasts, abdomen and perform any other special tests he feels necessary. He will also want to check your pelvic measurements to see if your pelvis is large enough to allow for a normal delivery.

In addition, he will want to weigh you, check your blood for Rh factor, your blood type and also to rule out venereal disease. This latter is required by law in most states. He will also test your blood to make sure you are not anemic.

## 1. Why Must I Have A Urine Specimen Each Time?

The doctor checks this for sugar to rule out diabetes, and for protein to be sure the kidney is functioning

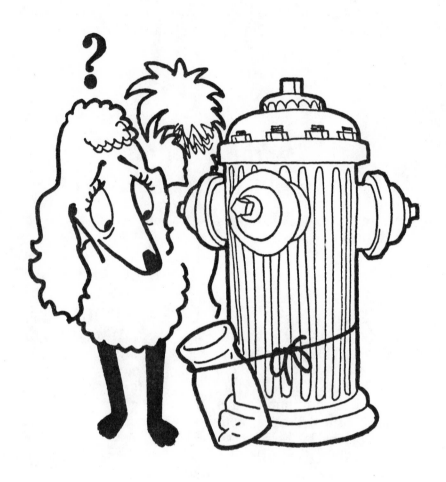

*Why Must I Have A Urine Specimen Each Time?*

normally as it eliminates your wastes. Also, he checks for bacteria and/or pus to make sure you don't have a urinary tract infection.

## 2. What About Diet In Pregnancy?

Previously, we have been anxious to limit a woman's weight in pregnancy in order to avoid toxemia of pregnancy, a condition characterized by increased weight gain, albumin in the urine and elevated blood pressure. However, it has been shown that adequate nutrition of the baby is more important. For this reason a woman's diet is restricted only as to excessive calories. She is allowed to eat a full diet to assure adequate nutrition for her baby.

## 3. What Is A Good Sample Diet To Follow?

An intake of about 2500 calories per day is adequate for the average woman.

She should have:

1. Protein—This to build good muscle tissue, skin, etc. A good source of protein is found in fish, chicken, meat, eggs, whole grain cereals, beans, and peas. About 85 grams of protein daily is desirable.

2. Carbohydrates—These should be eaten in restricted amounts, preferably no more than 150 grams daily.

3. Fat—These are energy foods and contain certain vitamins. But, these should be eaten sparingly.

4. Minerals—Calcium and phosphorus are used, not only by the mother, but also by the fetus for bone growth and development. A quart of milk per day insures an adequate amount of these.

Iron is easier to take as a tablet or capsule than trying to eat too many iron-rich foods. Iodine requirements can be met by eating one seafood per week.

5. Vitamins—These are best supplied by one multivitamin prenatal capsule per day.

43

## PROTEIN AND CALORIE CONTENT OF COMMON FOODS

| DAIRY FOODS | SIZE OF PORTION | Approx. PROTEIN (grams) | Approx. CALORIES |
|---|---|---|---|
| Milk, whole | 1 cup (8 oz.) | 9 | 160 |
| Milk, skimmed | 1 cup (8 oz.) | 9 | 90 |
| Cheese, American | 1 medium slice | 8 | 110 |
| Cheese, cottage, creamed | 2 tablespoons (1 oz.) | 4 | 30 |
| Cheese, cream | 2 tablespoons | 2 | 110 |
| Butter | 1 tablespoon | 6 | 100 |
| Cream, table | 2 tablespoons | 1 | 60 |
| Ice cream, vanilla | ¼ pint (½ cup) | 3 | 145 |

### MEAT, FISH, POULTRY, EGGS, LEGUMES

| | | | |
|---|---|---|---|
| Meat, lean | 1 ounce | 8 | 80 |
| Liver | 1 ounce | 8 | 65 |
| Bologna, frankfurter | 1 | 6 | 155 |
| Eggs | 1 egg, medium | 6 | 80 |
| Dried beans | ½ cup, cooked | 8 | 115 |
| Peanut butter | 2 tablespoons | 8 | 190 |
| Nuts | ½ cup peanuts | 19 | 420 |

### FRUITS

| | | | |
|---|---|---|---|
| Fresh, unsweetened | 1 medium serving | 1 | 50-100 |
| Cooked, lightly sweetened | ½ cup | 1 | 100 |

### VEGETABLES, COOKED

| | | | |
|---|---|---|---|
| Green, leafy | ½ cup | 2 | 20 |
| Root, as beets | ½ cup | 1 | 25 |
| Starchy, as corn | ½ cup | 3 | 85 |
| Potatoes, white | 1 medium | 2 | 80 |
| Legumes, young-peas, lima beans | ½ cup | 5-6 | 60-90 |

44

## BREADSTUFFS, CEREALS, PASTRIES

Bread, whole grain
or enriched ..............1 medium slice ............2 ............ 60
Cereal, cooked, whole
grain or enriched ........½ cup .....................2 ............ 60
Cereal, ready to eat
Whole grain or enriched .....¾ cup .....................1-2 ............ 80
Crackers, plain ...........2 crackers (medium) .......1 ............ 35
Cookies, plain ............2 small or 1 large .........1 ............ 120
Cake, not iced ............Med. Piece 2 x 3 x 1½" .....2 ............ 200
Cake, layer, icing .........Med. Piece 1/16 of 10" cake ..4 ............ 370
Pie, fruit ................1/7 medium ...............3 ............ 350
Pie, custard type ..........1/7 medium ...............8 ............ 280

## SAMPLE DIET

# BREAKFAST

| | |
|---|---|
| Fruit | Orange juice, ½ cup (4 oz.) |
| Cereal | Oatmeal, ½ cup |
| Bread and butter | Toast, 1 slice, butter, 1 tsp |
| Egg, if desired | One egg, cooked as you like (with 1 tsp. butter, if you wish) |
| Milk, to drink or with cereal | Milk, whole, 1 glass (8 oz.) |
| Coffee or tea | |

# LUNCH

| | |
|---|---|
| Main protein dish | Open-face broiled cheese sandwich; American cheese, 2 slices (2 oz.) |
| Bread and butter | Bread, 2 thin slices; butter, 1 tsp. |
| Vegetables | Salad, tomato and lettuce |
| Milk | Milk, whole, 1 glass (8 oz.) |
| Fruit | Grapefruit, half |

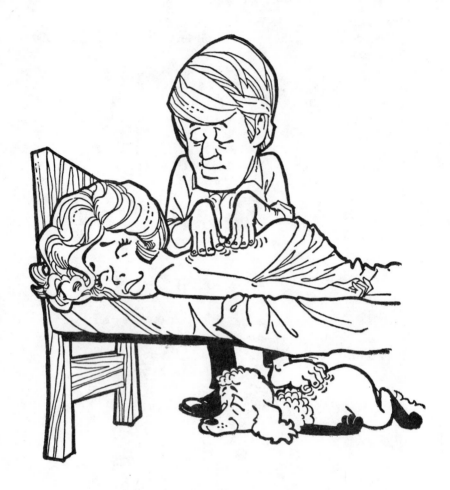

*What Can I Do For Backache In Pregnancy?*

## DINNER

Lean meat, fish, poultry, hamburger (3 oz. lean meat)
(or equivalent in protein)

Potato — Medium potato, baked
Other vegetables — Carrots, ½ cup
Butter — Butter for vegetables, 1-2 tsp.
Fruit or
  simple desert — Apple, medium


## BETWEEN MEALS

Fruit or Cheese

Your daily milk allowance can be taken
all or in part between meals if you wish.


### 4.  *What About Drugs In Pregnancy?*

One should take no unnecessary drug during pregnancy and none without the doctor's permission. Avoid hormones, antithyroid drugs and streptomycin. Streptomycin may cause hearing loss in the baby.

Tetracyclines (an antibiotic) may cause discoloration of the infant's teeth. Anticoagulants given for phlebitis may cause hemorrhage in the mother if given too close to delivery time.

Also—see Chapter 4, "Medicines in Pregnancy."


### 5.  *What Can I Do For Backache In Pregnancy?*

A firm mattress may help, along with heat and a back massage by your husband. You might also try better posture habits such as standing erect with even weight on each foot (some people stand on one foot, then the other). Flexing the knees while standing is also restful.

While sitting, most pregnant women find a straight-back chair is more comfortable. To keep from "slumping", tuck a small pillow at the small of your back. If your knees are lower than your hips, as you sit, elevate your feet by using a foot stool, or a stack of books, etc.

While lying on your back, place a pillow or folded blanket between your knees, under your abdomen, or along your back. If it becomes necessary to reach something from the floor or from a lower cupboard, you should squat down. This allows your legs to do the work, instead of putting a strain on your back.

### 6. Is Abdominal Pain More Serious In Pregnancy?

Just remember that even though you are pregnant, you can still have appendicitis, gall bladder attacks or other nonpregnancy related problems. If in doubt about abdominal pain, call your doctor.

Be aware, but not alarmed if your abdomen becomes firm, or if you experience more than ordinary discomfort— this could indicate labor. If in doubt, notify your doctor!

### 7. What Is Safe To Use For Constipation In Pregnancy?

This depends upon how severe the constipation is. However, there are a few simple things you might wish to try. For instance:
1. Increase the amount of water you drink to at least two quarts per day.
2. Certain fruits, such as prunes or other dried fruits, seem to help. Fruit juices may be just as effective.
3. Avoid harsh laxatives if possible.
4. In general, bulk laxatives or stool softeners are better than stronger laxatives. However, these cannot function unless taken with a large amount of water. They should not be taken unless ordered by your doctor.

48

5. Honey (one or two tablespoons) in a glass of warm water at night helps many women, and carries none of the disadvantages of other laxatives.

## 8. What Can I Do For Cramps In My Legs?

Calcium and vitamin D will help, as well as mild tranquilizers, especially if the cramps occur at night.

Leg cramps and charley horses at night are often caused from pointing your toes outward when you move or turn over. Use the reverse maneuver to rid you of the cramp, by bringing your toes toward your face and pushing out on your heels.

One or two tablespoons of honey in a glass of warm water have been found helpful by some women. Some think it acts as a muscle relaxant and also a mild sedative. Though the effect may be strictly psychological it may be worth trying and is not harmful.

A warm, (not hot), bath is also relaxing before you retire.

## 9. My Eyeglasses Seem Different Since I Became Pregnant. Do You Think I Should Have Them Changed?

For the most part, some refraction changes occur normally in pregnancy. For this reason, a change in glasses will not solve the problem for very long. Cut down on your reading, sewing, close eye-work, and watching television, to avoid eye strain.

Mild remedies such as aspirin usually will take care of most headaches. If possible defer getting new or different eyeglasses until after your pregnancy.

## 10. I Seem To Have So Much More Discharge When I Am Pregnant. Is This Normal?

Unless the discharge becomes truly troublesome, or

**49**

causes severe itching (often a sign of infection), it is normal and it can be ignored. But there is no need to put up with excessive discharge if it becomes uncomfortable. It can be treated and relieved by your doctor. Avoid self-treatment—leave the diagnosis and treatment to your doctor.

### 11. *I Have Never Fainted Before In My Life. Why Should I Have This During Pregnancy?*

Fainting sometimes goes along with a loss of tone in the muscle tissue that lines the blood vessels. This muscle tone is necessary to sustain blood pressure when the body position is changed.

In general, if you will take a little more time when you change positions, your body will adjust and you will be less likely to faint. Do not get up abruptly from a prone position—rather, roll to your side and then arise slowly.

If you feel as though you are going to faint, you should sit down, place your head between your legs, or lie down with your head lower than your body. If the faintness still persists, have someone raise your legs higher than your body. Usually this causes the blood to run to your head and you feel better almost immediately.

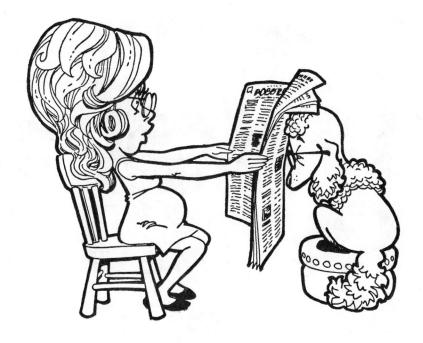

*My Eyeglasses Seem Different Since I Became Pregnant.
Do You Think I Should Have Them Changed?*

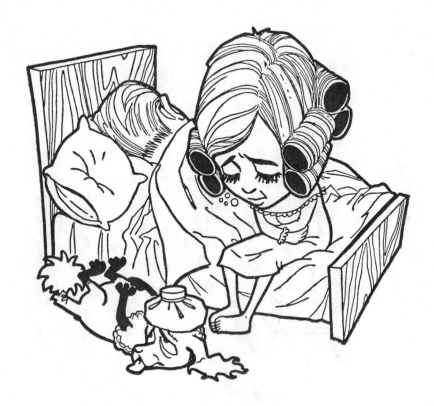

*Is Morning Sickness Really In A Woman's Head?*

# 5 | *Nausea And Vomiting Of Pregnancy*

### 1. *Is Morning Sickness Really In A Woman's Head?*

If it is, then over 60% of pregnant women have something wrong with their heads. Although everyone would concede a certain emotional element, it is unfair to say all nausea is in a woman's mind. Such statements usually come from men or from women who have never experienced the feeling. Nor is it limited to morning, although most women feel better as the day progresses.

### 2. *What Is The Cause Of Nausea And Vomiting Of Pregnancy?*

In addition to the emotional element, we think it has to do with certain hormones secreted during pregnancy. In addition to these causes, we find that digestion in general is slowed. Food often takes many, many hours to digest. In the meantime, it just "sits" there, as patients say, and produces a sensation of fullness and bloating. Sometimes diet plays an important role. In some women, it makes little difference what they eat . . . nothing digests well.

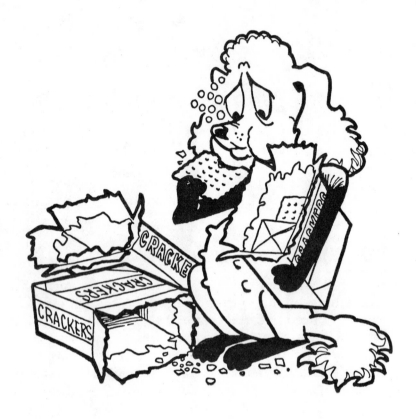

*What Can Be Done About Nausea Of Pregnancy?*

### 3. How Long Does Nausea And Vomiting Of Pregnancy Last?

Nausea may begin early in pregnancy and continue until your body adjusts to the vast amount of hormonal change. Ordinarily this takes about 12 weeks. Some fortunate people never experience nausea.

### 4. What Can Be Done About Nausea Of Pregnancy?

Much depends on how severe the nausea is. Some women have nausea just as they arise in the morning. For them the answer is to get rid of the early morning stomach residue by vomiting. After this they feel better, and often have no further nausea or vomiting for the remainder of the day.

Some very nervous women obtain great relief from a mild tranquilizer.

Certain women find it helpful to avoid fried or greasy foods, as well as rich desserts. Still others are helped by eating small, frequent meals that "keep something in the stomach". Crackers, melba toast, coke syrup, or thick cooked cereal are sometimes helpful. Most liquids taken while nauseated do not stay down.

For those who find no relief with such simple measures, a shot of vitamin B6 with or without vitamin B1 helps. Still others must be given anti-nauseants, by mouth if they can tolerate them. Anti-nauseants and barbiturates can also be given as a shot if the patient can get to the doctor's office. If not, the same medication may be given as rectal suppositories inserted by the patient.

### 5. What About Severe Cases of Nausea?

In extreme cases it may be necessary to hospitalize the patient, feed her intravenously, and regulate her electro-lyte balance (body chemicals) very carefully.

Only rarely is abortion necessary in these cases. It is

performed only for prolonged, persistent, or resistive nausea and vomiting of pregnancy.

### 6. If Nausea Is Severe With One Pregnancy, Does This Mean It Will Be Severe With The Next Pregnancy?

Not always, but often this is the case. Sometimes a tense home situation, marital difficulties, unwanted pregnancy, etc., tend to make the nausea more severe.

### 7. When Is Nausea And Vomiting Dangerous To A Pregnant Woman?

If nausea and vomiting persist, they cause alarming weight loss and a serious upset in the electrolyte balance in the body. The latter occurs because too much hydrochloric acid is lost from the stomach.

In severe cases, hospitalization becomes necessary but quickly overcomes the imbalance. Intravenous fluids and sedation help to correct the situation.

Unfortunately it is not uncommon to find that the nausea and vomiting recur after leaving the hospital. The symptoms subside after twelve to fourteen weeks of pregnancy.

# 6 | *Medicines In Pregnancy*

It is important that no unnecessary drugs be given in pregnancy. But it is just as important that necessary drugs not be withheld from the mother or fetus.

If you understand about drugs and pregnancy, you will also understand why your doctor gives you certain medicines and advises against other drugs during pregnancy.

### 1. *Do Most Women Take Medicines During Pregnancy?*

The average pregnant woman takes four or five different medicines during her pregnancy. About four out of five drugs taken by women in pregnancy are taken on their own, rather than by a doctor's prescription.

### 2. *Do All Of These Drugs The Mother Takes Pass Through To The Fetus?*

As far as we know, nearly *all* drugs pass through the placenta to the fetus in some amount. The so-called placental barrier between mother and baby is not a barrier to drugs.

### 3. Drugs Don't Cause All Of The Defects, Do They?

No. For instance, certain diseases such as German Measles cause defects. Heredity also plays an important role in defects. X-rays, certain industrial inhalants and other environmental factors can also cause defects.

### 4. How Early In A Pregnancy Can Drugs Pass Through The Placenta To The Fetus?

Generally speaking, drugs can pass freely either way through the placenta by the 5th week.

But *anytime* after conception the baby could be affected by drugs. Early in pregnancy, i.e. from conception to implantation (embedding) in the lining of the cavity of the uterus, a drug is likely to *kill* the embryo. After the 11th day it is more likely to cause a defect.

This could even occur before the mother had missed a menstrual period or was even aware that she was pregnant.

### 5. Are The Results Predictable?

Not always. The results are dependent upon many factors, including:
1. The type of drug.
2. The dose of the drug.
3. The time of gestation (how far along in pregnancy?)
4. The resistance or sensitivity of the fetus to particular drugs.

### 6. At What Period Of My Pregnancy Is My Baby Most Likely To Be Harmed By Drugs?

Usually during the first trimester (the first three

**59**

months) the fetus is most susceptible to drugs.

**7.** *Why Is The Period From The Third Week Of Pregnancy Through The Third Month Especially Important For The Fetus (As Far As Drugs Are Concerned?)*

This is the period of time during which the organs are formed and developing. During this time the cells are growing and multiplying rapidly and are therefore more sensitive to the effects of drugs.

**8.** *Does This Mean There Is No Danger From Drugs Taken After The First Three Months Of Pregnancy?*

No. There are certain drugs that still harm the baby during the second and third trimester (from the 4th through the 9th month of pregnancy). Your doctor understands these drugs and their actions. Take only the drugs he gives you and take them only as he directs you to take them.

**9.** *Can It Be Predicted Which Organ(s) Of The Baby Will Be Affected According To The Time In Pregnancy When The Drug Was Administered?*

Within certain limits this is possible.
In general:
The NERVOUS system is most likely to be harmed from the 15th to the 25th day.
The VISUAL system (eye) is most likely to be harmed from the 24th to the 40th day.
The HEART system is most likely to be harmed from the 20th to the 40th day.
The LEGS from the 24th to the 36th day of pregnancy.

60

## 10. How Do Drugs Cause Defects In The Fetus?

We don't know for sure. However there are several theories. For instance:

1. By reducing the oxygen-carrying capacity of the blood.
2. By reducing the amount of sugar in the blood.
3. By interfering with absorption of vitamins, hormones, and certain other vital substances.
4. By preventing the passage of oxygen across the placenta to the fetus.
5. By interfering directly with growth of the cells of the embryo.

## 11. What About Aspirin, Cold Tablets, Laxatives, Etc.?

The same rule applies. Whether tranquilizers, sedatives, antihistamines, weight control pills or pain pills, let your doctor decide. Sometimes drugs are very necessary to your health. Antibiotics, for instance, may be more important to control your infection, than any adverse effect they may have on your baby.

## 12. What Other Medicines Can I Take During Pregnancy?

A good general rule to follow is this: Take only those medicines that are prescribed by your doctor and only in the amounts he prescribes. Assume that all medicines pass through into your baby. Most are relatively harmless. Some are absorbed in only small amounts.

But all drugs must be weighed according to their need as well as to their effect upon the unborn baby. It is just as foolish to avoid a medicine that you need as it is to take one that you do not need. Let your doctor decide this for you.

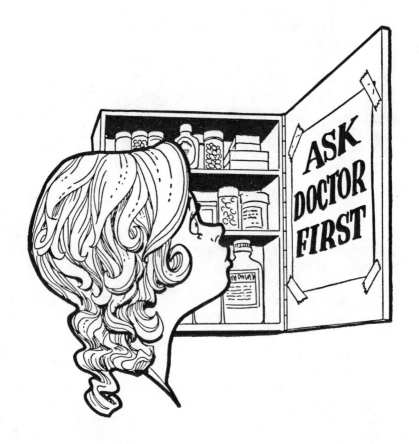

*What About Aspirin, Cold Tablets, Laxatives, Etc.?*

*REMEMBER—SOME DRUGS ARE LIFE-SAVING TO YOU AND TO YOUR BABY.*

But they must be taken properly—when and how they are prescribed by your doctor.

# 7 | What May I Do?

**1.** *Pregnancy Is Spoken Of As A "Delicate" Condition. What Am I Supposed To Avoid?*

Pregnancy is a normal physiological state. In general a woman may do anything during pregnancy that she does when she is not pregnant. There may be special circumstances in your particular pregnancy that require precautions, but a normal pregnancy is almost free of restriction as far as activity is concerned.

If you are used to tennis, golf, swimming, or bowling, for example, these sports will not harm you or your pregnancy. It is better not to undertake new and strenuous activities that overtax you or your strength. Be sure to discontinue any activity when you are tired.

**2.** *What About Bicycling, Horseback-Riding, And Skiing? Aren't These Too Vigorous For A Pregnant Woman?*

If a woman is accustomed to them and is in good physical condition they will not hurt her pregnancy.

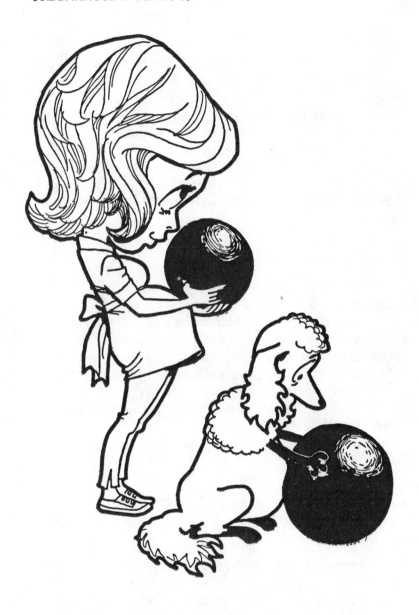

*Pregnancy Is Spoken Of As "Delicate" Condition.*
*What Am I Supposed To Avoid?*

65

However, she should know whether these sports are difficult for her even when she is pregnant.

Usually people are thinking of miscarriage when they ask such questions. A normal woman carrying a normal pregnancy is not likely to miscarry, regardless of her activity. Women have tried most means to abort an unwanted pregnancy, usually without success.

On the other hand, if there is something amiss with a pregnancy, a woman is likely to miscarry regardless of whether she remains in bed or is active. All sports or activities should be discontinued when the water breaks or the contractions are 5 minutes apart.

### 4. What About Climbing Stairs In Pregnancy?

Stairs are a good exercise for the average normal pregnant woman. If they prove to be too difficult for you, avoid them when possible. Sometimes a woman has excessive "relaxation" of her joints with a resultant loss of some support and stability. If this occurs in her hips, she may find it difficult to walk, let alone go up or down stairs.

A good rule to follow: never look at the stairs when you are going up or down. Before you start, look them over, then look straight ahead, keep your chin parallel to the stairs, then proceed up or down. Be sure to use the hand rail.

### 5. What About Swimming During Pregnancy? Will This Cause Infection?

Swimming is excellent exercise for pregnant women. Partly because of buoyancy, swimming is a less strenuous and a more relaxing sport than some others. There has been no evidence that it causes infection—other than athlete's foot if the woman is susceptible. Swimming is a good breast and chest exercise. Even the swimmer's breast stroke, done on "dry land", is beneficial.

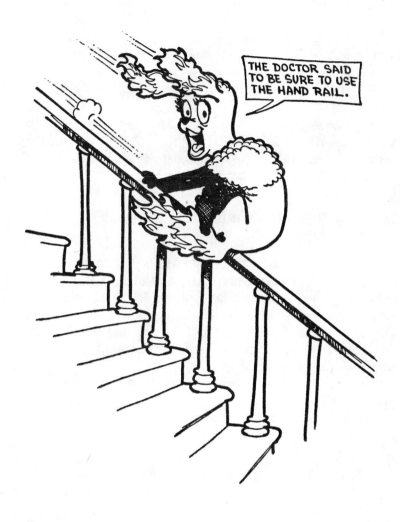

*What About Climbing Stairs In Pregnancy?*

### 6. What About X-Rays During Pregnancy? Will These Hurt The Baby?

The average x-ray pictures taken for diagnostic purposes do not subject the woman or the infant to a harmful dose. Naturally, it is better to avoid all x-rays unless they are absolutely necessary, especially during pregnancy.

However, it would be foolish to neglect an x-ray when it is necessary to diagnose a condition that might require important treatment. The radiologist will also "shield" the pregnancy from x-ray exposure if possible.

### 7. What About A Rubella (German Measles) Shot During Pregnancy?

These should never be given during pregnancy. Even when a woman is not pregnant, she should not have a Rubella shot unless she is willing to practice careful contraception for three months afterward. There is some slight chance that the attenuated (weakened) virus can get through to the fetus. The possibility of defects due to this is still under investigation.

Since 80% to 90% of women are already immune to Rubella, all women should have a test to determine this immunity before they are given a shot of the vaccine. This will avoid unnecessary shots.

### 8. How Dangerous Is It To Take The Birth Control Pill During Pregnancy? (By Mistake, Of Course)

Until we have longer experience with birth control pills, they are best not given during pregnancy. Nor should estrogens alone be given to pregnant women. There is some evidence that they have a tendency to cause cancer of the vagina (later on) in female babies born to these mothers.

68

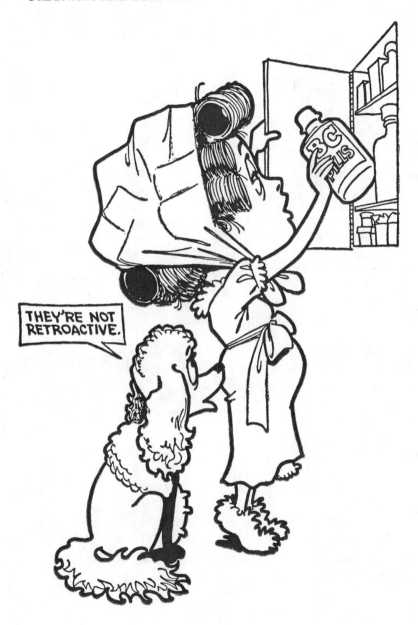

# 8 | The Rh Factor

### 1. What Does Rh Mean?

Rh is one of many substances called "factors" that are found in red blood cells. You might think of the Rh factor as covering the red blood cell like a coat of paint covers a golf ball.

### 2. How Common Is The Rh Factor?

There are several different Rh factors and everyone has some of these. The most important one is called the Rh "D" factor.

About 85% of all human beings have this coating which means that 15% do not have it. Those individuals who do not have this particular Rh factor are said to be "Rh negative."

### 3. Where Did The Name Come From?

It was named the Rh factor because it was originally discovered in the blood of *Rhesus* monkeys.

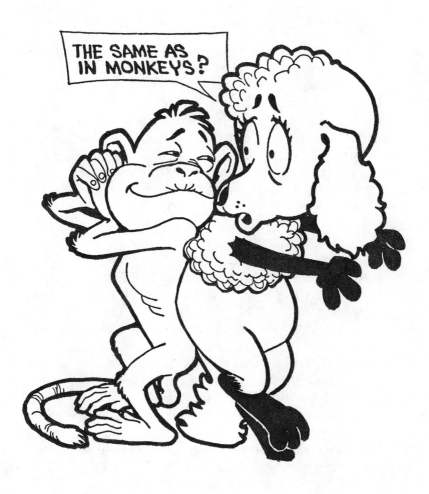

*Where Did The Name "RH" Come From?*
*From Rhesus Monkeys.*

## 4. Why Is The Rh Factor Important?

The chemical coating we call the Rh factor produces an "anti-body response" when introduced into the system of someone who does not have it. Antibodies are like reserve soldiers that are called out to protect the body against the intrusion of "foreigners." In this case the foreigners are the Rh-coated (Rh positive) red blood cells.

The body may tolerate a few foreigners, but if very many enter the blood stream (usually by way of a leak in the afterbirth) an alarm is sounded and the body's reserve troops (antibodies) are quickly produced.

This response becomes important in:

1. Transfusions:

Blood containing this factor (Rh-positive) is not given to people who do not have it (Rh-negative individual), because the person receiving the Rh-positive blood transfusion would then manufacture antibodies against the factor. This is called an "immune response" and the individual is then said to be "sensitized" against the Rh factor.

If an Rh-positive blood transfusion were given to this Rh-sensitized person, anti-Rh antibodies would be produced by the body just like nickels pouring from a jack-pot slot machine. The patient could suffer a very severe and possibly fatal reaction from this response.

2. Pregnancy:

Suppose an Rh-negative woman marries an Rh-positive man and they have an Rh-positive child. Ordinarily the blood of the fetus (the unborn child) does not come in contact with the blood of the mother. They have individual circulatory systems separated by a layer of tissue in the placenta (afterbirth).

However, if a small leak occurs in the placenta, allowing some of the baby's blood to enter the mother's circulatory system, the two incompatible bloods meet each other and conflict occurs similar to the above mentioned transfusion:

72

1. In the course of pregnancy (rarely happens),

2. During labor and delivery (occurs more often),

3. Or, immediately thereafter (occurs most commonly).

The result is that the mother (who does not have the Rh factor) treats the baby's blood (which *does* have the Rh factor) as a foreign element and this causes a "reaction."

The mother's Rh-negative blood responds to the baby's Rh-positive blood just as though it were a vaccination (like typhoid, polio, or Rubella) by producing antibodies against this substance (Rh factor coating around the baby's red blood cells).

This antibody response is part of the body's vital defense system (like a reserve army that quickly goes into action to protect its homeland from invasion by foreign agents), and is similar to the body's response to invasion by bacteria or viruses.

## 5. Why Is This Antibody Response Dangerous To The Baby?

Although the antibodies are produced for the protection of the mother, the mother has no way of controlling their effect upon the fetus. The fetus, in fact, is treated as an enemy of the mother.

These anti-Rh antibodies produced by the mother are small enough to pass freely through the placental barrier between the blood of the mother and that of the fetus. When these same anti-Rh antibodies reach the blood stream of the fetus they act like an army of retaliation. The result is that they DESTROY the baby's Rh-positive red blood cells.

In an effort to compensate for this loss, the fetus speeds up its production line and turns out INCOMPLETELY FORMED red blood cells (like immature, poorly-trained troops), called ERYTHROBLASTS. From

73

this process comes the name of the disease—ERYTHRO-BLASTOSIS FETALIS (incompletely developed red blood cells produced by the fetus).

This process may be compared to a production line in a factory that turns out hastily and poorly assembled automobiles that never function the way they should.

### 6. Is There Any Way To Tell How Severe The Disease Is Or How Much It Is Affecting The Fetus?

Yes. By inserting a needle through the mother's abdominal wall, through the uterus and finally penetrating the thin amniotic sac surrounding the baby (called amniocentesis), some of this amniotic fluid can be withdrawn and examined in the laboratory.

The tests performed upon this fluid will tell us how severe the destruction of the baby's blood is. It is almost like looking through a telescope to see how the battle is progressing;

1. If The Pregnancy Is Close To The Normal Time For Delivery—

It may be allowed to continue, if the involvement is not too severe. After delivery the baby's blood can be replaced a little at a time, by withdrawing some of the baby's blood, then replacing it with equal amounts of normal blood and repeating this process. This is called an EXCHANGE TRANSFUSION. In this manner normal blood is exchanged for the damaged blood of the baby.

2. If The Test On The Amniotic Fluid Surrounding The Fetus Shows Destruction Of The Infant's Blood Is Too Severe To Wait And If The Baby Is Not Too Premature—

The baby can be delivered early (to avoid further damage). After delivery it is immediately given one or more exchange transfusions. If the process has not progressed too far and the damage to the baby is not too great, these babies can be saved by the transfusions.

3. If The Baby Is Too Premature For Delivery—

The fetus can be given a blood transfusion while it is still in the uterus. To accomplish this a special needle is inserted through the mother's abdomen and uterus and into the baby's abdominal cavity where normal red blood cells are deposited for absorption and use by the baby. Some babies require several of such transfusions to keep them alive until they are mature enough to survive at delivery.

### 7. Is There Anything That Can Be Done To Prevent Rh Sensitization In The Mother?

Yes. If the mother can be given "ready-made" anti-Rh antibodies with which to combat the invading Rh-positive (coated baby's red blood cells which enter her blood through a break in the placenta at the time of delivery) she will not have to manufacture her own antibodies. This is called "passive" immunity. But this immunity is temporary and the ready-made antibodies disappear after a few weeks (similar to giving a person tetanus antitoxin to prevent lockjaw (tetanus) when she steps on a rusty nail).

If sensitization in the mother is thus prevented, she will not produce anti-Rh antibodies which would destroy the red blood cells of the next Rh-positive baby the mother might have. In other words, erythroblastosis is prevented before it has a chance to develop.

This is similar to importing mercenary soldiers to handle a temporary emergency. They are no longer needed when the emergency is over. After their job is done, they leave the country.

75

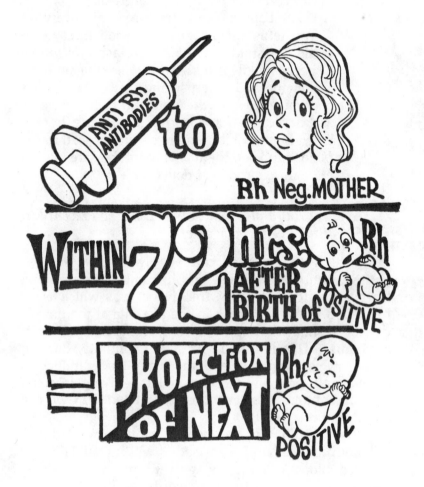

*Is There A Shot That Will Give The Mother This Passive Immunity?*

## 8. Is There A Shot That Will Give The Mother This Passive Immunity?

Yes. There is an hyperimmune gamma globulin which provides "ready-made" anti-Rh antibodies. If it is given within 72 hours of birth of an Rh-positive infant, it will give the Rh-negative mother an "unsensitized" passive immunity.

## 9. Where Do The Antibodies Come From That Are Found In the Hyperimmune Gamma Globulin?

These are human anti-Rh antibodies obtained from people (recruited mercenaries) who have developed an ACTIVE immunity against the RH factor.

## 10. How Long Does This Passive Immunity Last?

Probably only for a few weeks, but this is the period during which sensitization occurs. If a non-sensitized Rh-negative mother has an injection of immune anti-Rh antibodies immediately after each Rh-positive baby, the next baby will be protected against erythroblastosis.

### Summary

1. Rh is a chemical coating found on the red blood cells of 85% of human beings. These individuals are said to be "Rh positive," which means that the remaining 15% who do not have it are "Rh-negative."
2. The Rh factor can provoke an immune reaction if it gets into the blood stream of a person who does not have this factor. This is called sensitization.
3. Sensitization becomes important in transfusions and pregnancy because it can result in severe reactions or even death of the person or in an unborn baby.
4. The problem can be eliminated in transfusions by

never giving Rh-positive blood to Rh-negative individuals.

5. Already-sensitized pregnant women must be treated by:

    a. Early delivery of the baby in some cases.

    b. Exchange transfusions of babies immediately after birth in others.

    c. Intra-uterine transfusions of the fetus in those severe cases in which the baby is too premature to be delivered.

6. Most non-sensitized Rh-negative mothers can be protected against sensitization by providing "passive immunity" against the Rh factor. This is done by giving them hyperimmune gamma globulin within 72 hours after the birth of every Rh-positive child. This protects the next Rh-positive child against erythroblastosis.

# 9 | Rubella (German Measles) During Pregnancy

This disease has been called "German" measles since the early 1800's because a German scientist pointed out the differences between this disease and regular measles, scarlet fever, and a few other diseases. It is neither German nor measles.

### 1. What Is The Incubation Period Of Rubella?

Normally 2 to 3 weeks after exposure. The exposed person can spread the disease even if he shows NO symptoms.

### 2. What Are The Symptoms?

All or none of these symptoms may occur—light rash, slightly raised temperature, some swelling of the neck, general discomfort, headache, sore throat, redness of the eyes and loss of appetite. If any of these symptoms appear at all, they last only about 3 days.

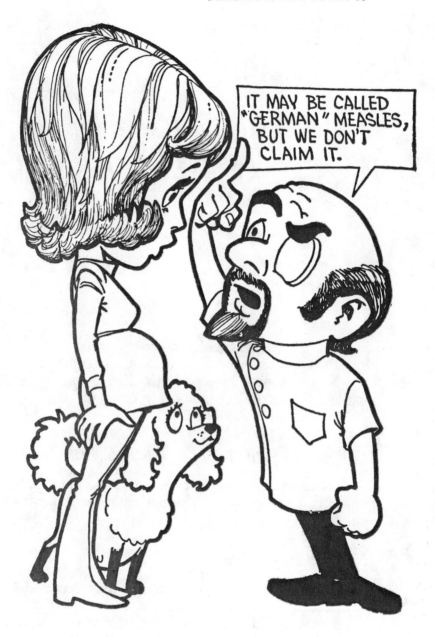

*What Is The Incubation Period Of Rubella?*

### 3. If I Had Rubella, How Long Could I Infect Others?

Contagion is possible for at least 2 weeks after the rash appears, or for 4 to 6 weeks after the original exposure. (Note: some evidence indicates an infected person can continue to spread the disease for months afterwards.)

### 4 Would My Doctor Be Able To Tell Me If I Have Rubella For Sure?

The diagnosis cannot be based on symptoms, which are often irregular, minimal, or even non-existent. Accurate diagnosis is possible only by isolation of the virus from body tissues, or by blood tests. In the last epidemic, many infected infants were born to mothers totally unaware that they had rubella during pregnancy.

A new technique, the HI test, can test blood within several hours and detect immunity years after the infection. The State Health Department Lab can perform this test. Because facilities are still limited, it is not yet possible to offer HI testing as a regular service in all states.

### 5. What Is The Treatment Of Rubella?

Unless a complication occurs, rubella seldom requires any treatment beyond the customary rest and recuperation. Complications are not as common as are complications in measles, but they did appear with some frequency in the 1964 epidemic.

### 6. Why Is Rubella So Dangerous For Pregnant Women?

Rubella produces few if any symptoms in the mother, but it may be readily passed on to the fetus. Here it causes either death in the fetus or defects in a large percentage of them.

For instance, in the epidemic of 1964, it was estimated that about 20,000 babies were born in the United States with severe birth defects, and an estimated 30,000 others died. This, of course, was before vaccine was available.

### 7. What Defects Does Rubella Cause?

The most frequent defects are:

1. Hearing loss. Unless it is in the form of virtual deafness, as is often the case, the loss of hearing may not be discovered until the child reaches school age.

2. Vision loss. This includes blindness. Most common defects are cataracts, glaucoma, abnormally small eyeball-size, defects of the retina, and clouding of the cornea.

3. Heart defects. Sometimes these are not apparent at birth. They become a frequent cause of death during early infancy.

4. Abnormalities of the central nervous system. This includes brain damage which results in cerebral palsy, and in mental retardation. Another common deformity is abnormally small head size.

### 8. How Can I Know If I Have Rubella During Pregnancy?

You can't, really. You may develop a mild pink rash and some fever, but there are many other diseases that produce these same symptoms. The only way you can be certain is to have a blood test for the disease

### 9. What Should I Do Then, To Protect My Future Pregnancies Against Rubella?

We now have a vaccine that will protect you against the development of rubella.

## 10. *Should Everyone Be Vaccinated?*

No, for several reasons. First of all, by the age of 11, about 80% of the population has had rubella and therefore has a natural immunity against the disease. By the age of 20, about 92% of the population has been immunized in the same manner.

First of all, we must identify those who are not immune and see that they are immunized. This can be determined by a blood test. Those who are immune need no treatment or precautions.

## 11. *What If I Am Already Pregnant?*

You should not be immunized. Although we think there is no danger or damage to your baby, we have not had the vaccine long enough to be sure. Therefore, pregnant women should not receive the vaccine.

## 12. *What If I Am Not Sure If I Am Pregnant Or Not?*

Don't take the vaccine. If it is given to an adult woman of child-bearing age, it should be given right after her menstrual period and only if she is willing to take birth control precautions for at least three months.

## 13. *What About Immunization Of Children?*

Yes, by all means. Beginning at one year (after natural immunity has worn off) and up to age 9 is the most susceptible time. After these ages are immunized, a continuous program of immunization of all two year-olds would gradually eliminate the menace.

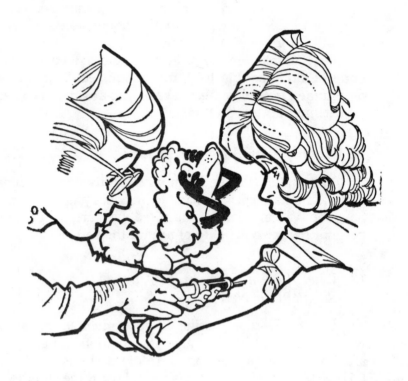

*Should Everyone Be Vaccinated Against German Measles?*
*Not If Immune Or Pregnant.*

## 14. What About Rubella Parties, In Which Children Are Exposed To Measles To Immunize Them?

This is definitely not recommended because there are some serious complications, though rare, to rubella. One of these is rubella encephalitis, in which the disease may produce permanent damage, including mental retardation and even death.

Such an epidemic of measles may also expose more pregnant women to the disease.

## 15. Should A Woman Be Aborted If She Develops Rubella In Pregnancy?

This is, of course, up to her and her doctor. However, the education of a blind child costs $10,000 per year plus $3,000 custodial care—with lifetime cost estimated at $340,000, to say nothing of the heartache to the child and parents.

Frustration in children over this defect causes anxieties, rages, and tantrums that place threatening stresses upon the home and the marriage. Rubella is a home wrecker.

But there are also other less common (but serious) defects and damage produced by the rubella virus in the unborn child. Some of these are:

1. Stunted growth. Many of the babies weighed less than five pounds at birth. After birth, many had feeding problems and gained weight very slowly.
2. Purple "birth marks." These reddish or purplish spots—sometimes called "wine-stains"—are particularly found on the face. They are caused by a bleeding tendency associated with low blood platelets (the blood's natural clotting agent).

But any decision regarding abortion should be left strictly up to the mother.

# 10 | Husbands And Pregnancy

### 1. My Husband Seems To Love Me Even More Now That I Am Pregnant, But I Am Afraid We Might Harm The Baby, Are There Any Restrictions?

I assume you mean in love-making. No, there are no restrictions unless such love-making is painful (it shouldn't be), or distasteful (if it is, check with your doctor to find out what your hang-up is).

Intercourse during pregnancy is normal and even beneficial for both husband and wife. Frequently husband and wife feel closer at this time than at any other time during their entire marriage.

### 2. Will Intercourse Make Me Miscarry?

No. There is no evidence to show that it will. If intercourse will cause you to miscarry, then many other ordinary activities would also do so. If a woman is threatening to miscarry, there is a possibility that miscarriage could occur, but even so, the die is usually

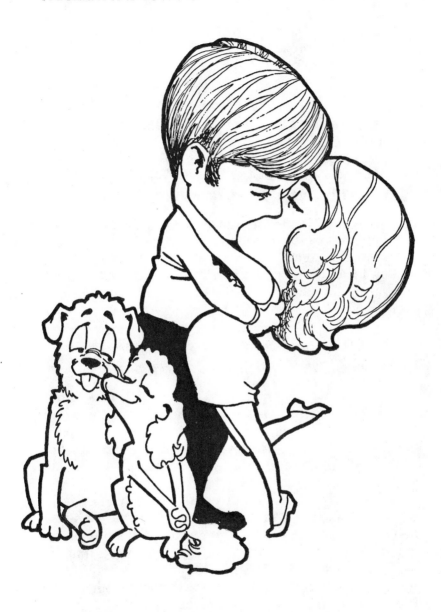

*My Husband Seems To Love Me Even More Now That I Am Pregnant, But I Am Afraid We Might Harm The Baby. Are There Any Restrictions?*

cast. If the pregnancy is normal, a woman will usually carry it. If the pregnancy is abnormal, she will usually lose it regardless of what she does.

**3.** *When I Am Trying To Conceive, Our Love-Making Seems To Take On A New And Greater Dimension. We Seem To Be "One Flesh" As They Say. I Just Can't Describe How Marvellous It Is. How Can I Make My Husband (And Myself) Feel This Ecstatic Feeling At Other Times, Too?*

Emotions play a great role in sex as your observation proves. Perhaps this demonstrates to you that you CAN enjoy sex this much on other occasions, too, if—you are willing to set the stage, put forth the effort, and make of sex a truly fulfilling experience for both of you. It can be done!

**4.** *Should A Husband Be Allowed In The Delivery Room At The Time His Wife Has Her Baby?*

Do you want him there? Do hospital rules permit him to be there? There are many advantages to having the father participate and share this marvellous experience with his wife. However, some husbands do not wish to be there, and others, because of their attitude and behavior, should not be there.

If a husband can be given some orientation as to what will take place in the delivery room and what role he should play, he can be a comforting influence for his wife at this time. Most men prefer standing or sitting by her side to give her support in his own way. Most women prefer to have the husband there, rather than further away from her—"looking on."

**5.** *Is It Normal To Dislike Sex During Pregnancy?*

No. This usually stems from a subconscious fear of

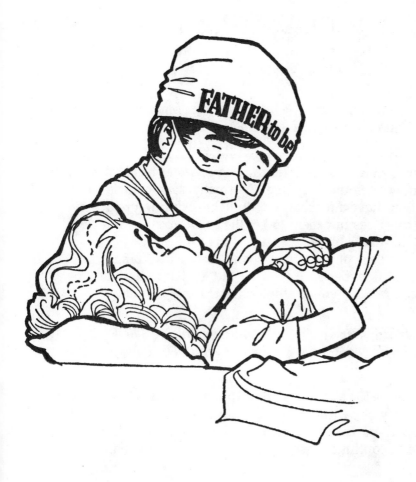

*Should A Husband Be Allowed In The Delivery Room At The Time His Wife Has Her Baby?*

harming the baby, something that simply does not occur. If you cannot overcome this fear, discuss it with your doctor. He can usually reassure you and help you to overcome any fears that are unwarranted.

Most couples enjoy sex more during pregnancy because the problem of birth control is eliminated. During most pregnancies they feel closer to each other.

### 6. Is There Danger Of Infection From Intercourse, Especially Toward The End Of Pregnancy?

No. There has been no evidence to show that this occurs, unless, of course, the bag of water has broken or if there is some bleeding. Normally a woman is more likely to have a discharge with itching during pregnancy, but this does not seem to be due to intercourse, nor does it affect the baby.

Occasionally both husband and wife "ping-pong" an infection back and forth, but this infection can be diagnosed and effectively treated during pregnancy.

### 7. Is It Better To Avoid Intercourse During The First Three Months Of Pregnancy While The Baby Is Forming?

No. This is a time when husband and wife should feel very close to each other. Since we have no proof of harm done by intercourse during pregnancy, it seems wise to continue it as though she were not pregnant.

### 8. But Surely We Should Stop Having Intercourse During The Last Six Or Eight Weeks Of Pregnancy, Shouldn't We?

Do you want to? There is no medical reason that you should. If it becomes too uncomfortable for the wife in the latter stages of pregnancy, they can use a little

90

ingenuity, try other positions, etc., and still continue relations.

If the wife is especially protuberant, the husband may find he can enter the vagina from the rear, causing little or no discomfort for his wife. If the husband is gentle, and the wife is not uncomfortable, sex should be enjoyed until the bag of water breaks or the contractions are five minutes apart.

### 9. Can A Woman Still Have An Orgasm Even Though She Is Pregnant?

Many women find their libido and satisfaction greatly heightened during pregnancy, perhaps because they do not have to worry about becoming pregnant. Sometimes fatigue interferes. Occasionally a woman feels "unlovely" (not true).

But generally speaking, sex should continue unabated during pregnancy. A thoughtful husband will help his wife, by digital clitoral stimulation, when necessary, to achieve orgasm during pregnancy.

If a woman is prone to miscarriage or premature delivery, she may have to forego orgasm (not inter course) during the first three months of pregnancy or during the last two months of pregnancy. In some women, orgasm provokes painful uterine contractions that could lead to miscarriage or early labor.

### 10. Is There Any Reason That Nipple Stimulation (During Intercourse) Should Be Discontinued During Pregnancy?

No, unless this is distasteful to either partner.

# 11 | *Danger Signs Of Pregnancy*

*1. Are There Any Special Danger Signs I Should Look For In Pregnancy?*

Yes. Occasionally a baby decides to complicate its mother's life even before it is born. There are a few tricks a baby may try which cause symptoms your doctor will want to know about as soon as they occur. These symptoms do not necessarily spell trouble. Rather they indicate that some treatment may be in order to ward off trouble. Call your doctor if any of these symptoms appear:

a. *Bloody Discharge From The Vagina.* Early in pregnancy this could mean a threatened miscarriage, or later on it could mean:

1) The afterbirth is in front of the baby.

2) Separation of the afterbirth before labor.

3) The onset of labor.

In the first part of pregnancy, if the bleeding is just staining (less than normal menstrual flow) the news will keep until morning. But in the second half

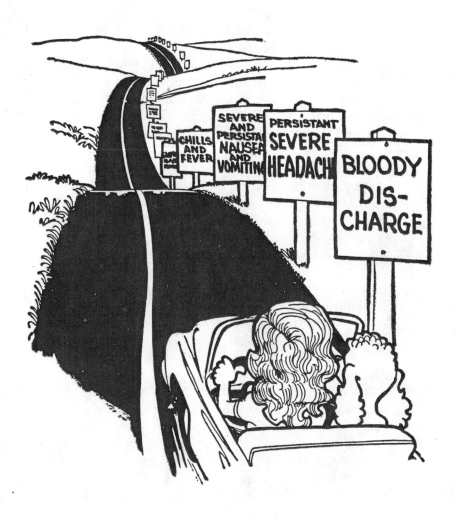

CHILLS AND FEVER

SEVERE AND PERSISTANT NAUSEA AND VOMITING

PERSISTANT SEVERE HEADACH

BLOODY DIS-CHARGE

*Are There Any Special Danger Signs
I Should Look For In Pregnancy?*

93

of pregnancy notify the doctor day or night, irrespective of the amount of bleeding. This does not include pink, mucoid discharge at term ("show").

b. *Persistent Severe headaches.* These can indicate toxemia of pregnancy, high blood pressure, or in rare cases, a brain tumor.

c. *Severe And Persistent Nausea and Vomiting.* This is discussed in the chapter on nausea and vomiting. However, when there is vomiting several times within a few hours, it is a danger sign and should be reported immediately to your doctor.

d. *Chills And Fever Of Over 100 Degrees, Other Than With A Common Cold.* High fever can injure or even destroy a fetus. Hence, a high fever, particularly associated with a chill, should be reported immediately to your doctor.

e. *Swelling Of The Ankles, Feet, Hands, And Face.* This can be an indication of toxemia of pregnancy and should be reported. Puffiness of the face, eyes, or fingers are particularly significant if very sudden. Swelling of the legs and ankles when the face and hands are uninvolved may not be significant, especially in hot weather.

f. *Severe Abdominal Pain.* Unless it is a momentary catch, or associated with constipation, report abdominal pain to your doctor. Remember that pregnant women can also have appendicitis, gall bladder attacks, etc.

g. *Sudden Gush Of Water From The Vagina.* This could indicate the opening of the membranes, resulting in the uncontrolled escape of watery fluid. When this "bag of waters" is broken, labor usually ensues, regardless of the duration of the pregnancy.

h. *Frequent, Burning Urination.* This usually indicates a bladder infection. By reporting this to your doctor you can obtain early and effective relief from the symptoms as well as the cure of the infection.

i. *Reduced Amount Of Urine, With Or Without Increased*

94

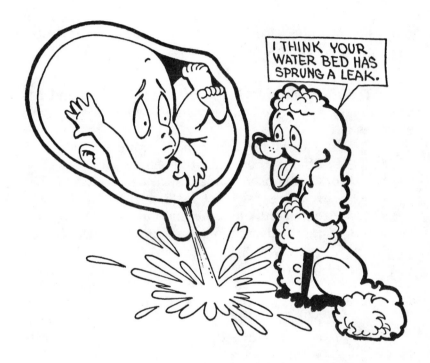

*Sudden Gush Of Water From The Vagina.*

*Thirst.* If you are thirsty, your doctor will check you for diabetes. If no diabetes is found, decreased amount of urine could still be a serious sign and you should be checked by your doctor to rule out any kidney trouble.

j. *Dimness Or Blurring Of Vision.* This is especially important in the second half of pregnancy.

**2.** *I Hate To Bother My Doctor. In General, What Are Some Of The Rules I Should Follow About Calling Him?*

There are times when you *should* call him and he would want you to call him. BUT—here are a few suggestions:

    (a) Except for emergencies, phone him at his office rather than at his home.

    (b) Don't play games such as asking if he remembers you. Instead, give him your name and any other helpful information, the fact you are pregnant, how far along, and when you were last in his office.

    (c) If you cannot telephone the doctor yourself, be sure to have the person making the call well informed about the details. For instance, if the condition prompting the call is vaginal bleeding in pregnancy, you must let him know:

        1. How much blood is being passed.

        2. Is it mere spots or streaks mixed with mucous?

        3. How does it compare with the first day of a menstrual period? Is it more or less?

        4. Has there been any pain associated with the bleeding? If so, is it in the midline and cramp-like in character, or is it on one side or the other of the abdomen?

(d) If your bag of water has broken, be sure to tell him of this.

(e) If reporting uterine contractions—how often? How long do they last? How severe? Any bearing down sensations?

(f) If reporting about your urinary tract, are you passing blood—how much—how often are you urinating—how painful—any pain in your back?

(g) Talk to the doctor yourself if at all possible. To relay questions and answers back and forth through a third party is not only likely to result in a misleading story for the doctor, and garbled advice for you, but trebles the time consumed by the call. Have a pencil and paper handy in case you must write down instructions.

(h) When calling your doctor, it is good to know the name, address, and telephone number of your nearest pharmacy. Your doctor may wish to telephone a prescription for you, and it will obviously expedite matters if you can give this information.

# 12 | *Some Normal Discomforts Of Pregnancy*

### 1. *Is It Normal To Be Fatigued All The Time?*

To some women, this is the first indication that they may be pregnant. In many, the basal metabolism is slowed during the first three months of pregnancy. Your doctor will determine if you need thyroid medicine or not.

Don't be worried if you require considerably more sleep than you did before pregnancy. A wise expectant will sneak in a nap or two during the day. Those who *never* get enough sleep can simply be happy they aren't elephants—who have a three year gestation period for each pregnancy.

If fatigue is out of all proportion, tell your doctor so he can check further on your blood and make any additional tests he feels are necessary.

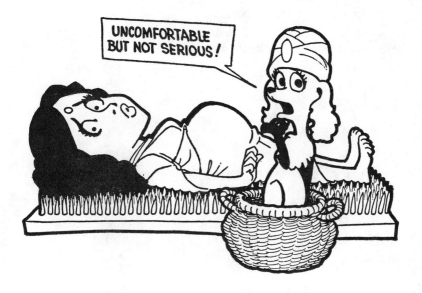

*There Are Certain Symptoms In Pregnancy That Are More Uncomfortable Than They Are Serious.*

Sometimes, a small amount of fatigue is necessary to slow you down while you are pregnant.

## 2. Why Doesn't My Food Digest?

Digestion is slowed and often food feels as though it just "sits there" like a lump in your stomach. However, you should try the following:
1. Antacids may help.
2. Learn what agrees with you and what does not. Then eat accordingly.
3. Eat small meals, eat more often, and chew your food well.
4. Discontinue fried, greasy foods and rich pastries.

Most women find that digestion returns to normal after the pregnancy.

## 3. I Have Never Had Constipation Before—Why Now?

Constipation is related to indigestion in pregnancy. The "tone" of the bowel muscles is diminished and the bowel simply does not do its job as it should. Prune juice, orange juice, and increased liquids in general seem to help.

Avoid harsh laxatives altogether, as well as repeated enemas. Usually a bulk laxative that also acts as a stool softener will answer your needs.

## 4. Why Do I Have So Much Backache All Of A Sudden?

The ligaments of the body seem to lose much of their tone and apparently relax. As a result they do not support your joints as they should. This is most noticeable in joints that bear weight such as in your pelvis and back.

Pregnant women walk with their legs farther apart to compensate for this poor support and to retain their balance. They also have more pain in their back and hips because of this lack of support.

### 5. What Can I Do For This Backache?

Correcting your posture often helps, but occasionally a brace or pelvic support is necessary, especially during the last few months of pregnancy.

Low-heel shoes generally "feel" more comfortable. Standing on your feet too long may bring on discomfort and fatigue sooner during pregnancy.

Most pregnant women have more backache if their mattress is soft or "saggy." Before you purchase a new mattress, try a factory-made bed board or a wide piece of plywood under your present mattress.

Pain relieving drugs should be taken only when prescribed by your doctor.

### 6. Why Do I Have To Urinate More Often?

Early in pregnancy the enlarging uterus compresses the bladder. After three or four months this symptom is relieved as the uterus rises out of the pelvis, only to return later when the baby's head descends into the pelvis and once more presses on the bladder.

This frequency of urination is not an indication of bladder infection. It is simply one of the expected discomforts and inconveniences of pregnancy.

You may want to limit your fluids after your evening meal to insure a longer, less-interrupted sleep.

### 7. Why Do I Cry So Easily?

A pregnant woman's feelings are more fragile and she typically may cry easily, often, and frequently without justifiable provocation. This calls for understanding on the part of your husband and both of you must realize that this is temporary and not serious.

**101**

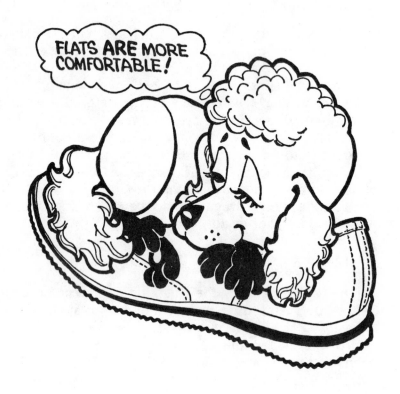

*What Can I Do For My Backache?*

## 8.  Why Do I Faint So Easily?

The tone of the muscles lining the blood vessels is decreased during pregnancy. If you stand on your feet too long, when you enter a warm room, or when you get too tired you may faint. Sudden changes of position (such as rising quickly from your bed) may cause you to faint, or at least to "feel faint."

Rapid relief is obtained by lowering your head—placing it between your knees if sitting, or preferably by lying down. Raising your legs above your body brings relief even more quickly.

Do not drink water, especially if you are only partially awake and alert. Never pour water into the mouth of a person who has fainted.

## 9.  Why Does My Skin Feel So Tight?

Your skin may be stretching, but it is not uncommon to feel as though it is tightly stretched during pregnancy. Have your husband massage your skin gently with a lotion. It won't prevent stretch marks, but at least it will make you feel better.

# 13 | *Vaginal Discharge In Pregnancy*

Many women will have a vaginal infection at some time during their pregnancy, regardless of personal cleanliness. Nor is infection limited to any race, age, or social standing.

Although difficult to completely cure during pregnancy, most infections can be controlled and the symptoms relieved. However, since there are different types of infection, each with its own specific treatment, the type of infection must first be determined before it can be successfully treated.

### 1. Is It Normal To Have A Vaginal Discharge?

Yes. Normally there is a clear secretion from the cervical glands. As this secretion proceeds down the vaginal tract it joins with discarded cells from the walls of the vagina, which cause it to become whitish and cloudy.

This type of discharge is normal. It does not require any hygienic measures other than normal bathing and

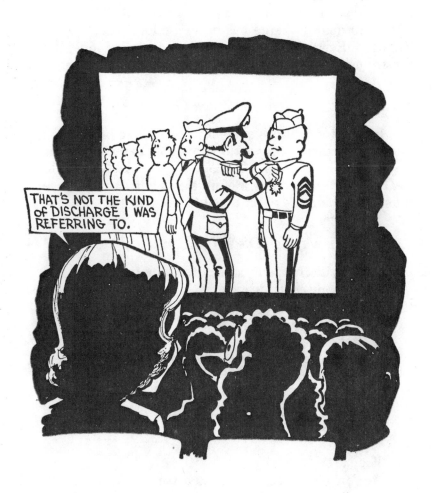

*Is It Normal To Have A Vaginal Discharge?*

personal cleanliness. Douches and medications are not necessary; in fact, they may be harmful if used to "cure" a normal discharge.

A normal discharge has no foul odor and causes no irritation. Every woman has some vaginal discharge, but the amount may vary according to the individual.

## 2. Where Does Vaginal Infection Originate?

Except for that of venereal infection, we often don't know the sources, but we do know how to recognize the cause and the type of infection. We also know how to treat the different types. Before treatment, however, we must determine the exact type of infection.

## 3. When Is Vaginal Discharge Considered Abnormal?

Vaginal discharge is considered abnormal:
A. If it causes itching.
B. If it causes swelling.
C. If it causes irritation.
D. If it causes an unpleasant odor.
E. If it becomes so excessive that it is annoying to the patient.

## 4. What Are The Most Common Types Of Vaginal Infection?

They are:
A. Parasitic infection due to a parasite called Trichomonas vaginalis.
B. Fungus infection due to a yeast-like fungus called Monilia albicans.
C. Bacterial infection due to various bacteria (most commonly the haemophilus vaginalis).

106

5. *Do The Various Infections Cause Similar Symptoms?*

Yes. For the most part all of them cause the following symptoms:
   A. Itching
   B. Irritation.
   C. Swelling of vaginal tissue.
   D. Odorous discharge.

6. *Does The Vaginal Discharge Look The Same In Each Type of Infection?*

No. Each type usually has its own typical appearance. For example:
   A. Trichomonal infection produces a greenish-yellow, foamy type of vaginal discharge.
   B. Monilial (yeast-like fungus) infection produces a thick, white, curd-like vaginal discharge that clings to the walls of the vagina and the cervix.
   C. Bacterial infection may vary, but usually it causes a vaginal discharge that is watery and full of pus.

7. *How Can A Woman Be Sure Which Type Of Infection She Has?*

Only her physician can tell. By pelvic and microscopic examination, however, he can determine the type of discharge. He will then prescribe the specific treatment necessary.

8. *Is It Possible To Have More Than One Type of Infection?*

Yes. This is called a "mixed" infection. A woman could have any two or even all three types of infection at the same time. This could account for the fact that occasionally a woman does not respond to a specific treatment. The treatment used may be designed to clear up one type of infection, while leaving the other infection unchecked.

**9. Are There Other Causes Of Irritation And Discharge Beside These Infections?**

Yes. For instance:

A. Diabetes can cause vaginal irritation with or without vaginal discharge. It can be diagnosed by urine and blood tests.

B. Birth control pills (naturally not a problem in pregnancy) often cause an increased amount of discharge. Yeast infection is more common in women taking birth control pills.

C. Antibiotics. Certain antibiotics often kill off the bacteria which are natural antagonists to fungus infections and serve to keep fungi under control. When these bacteria are eliminated by an antibiotic, fungi may grow unchecked.

D. Nervousness may cause an increase in the amount of normal vaginal discharge!

E. Venereal disease. Gonorrheal infection may look like any other bacterial infection. It must be diagnosed by a physician. It can be effectively treated with antibiotics.

**10. Is It Normal To Have Increased Vaginal Discharge During Pregnancy?**

Yes, in most cases. The tissues of the cervix and vagina are more congested with blood during pregnancy and it is also common to have some erosion (irritation) of the cervix. Both of these factors seem to increase the amount of discharge.

108

### 11. Is Vaginal Infection Injurious To A Pregnant Woman Or Her Baby?

Trichomonal or bacterial infection is usually more annoying than injurious. "Thrush," a fungus infection of the mouth, occasionally develops in the baby when the mother has a vaginal fungus (yeast) infection. This is easily treated and leaves no harmful after-effect. However, an infection can be injurious to the baby and the mother if due to venereal infection.

### 12. Is Treatment The Same For All Types Of Vaginal Discharge?

Obviously not. After diagnosis, specific treatment for that particular type of infection must be carried out. For treatment to be effective, however, it should be used exactly as prescribed by your physician!

### 13. Is The Infection Cured When The Symptoms Disappear?

Often not. The infection is cured only after all of the causative organisms are gone. Only your physician can determine this and only by examination.

### 14. Can Vaginal Infections Be Treated Just The Same During Pregnancy As In The Non-Pregnant State?

No. There are certain antibiotics which should not be used during pregnancy. For instance, tetracyclines may discolor the baby's teeth.

### 15. Avoid Self-Medication For Vaginal Infections!

Call your doctor's attention to your problem. He will then determine the cause of your infection and outline a complete treatment program for you. Your husband may also have to be treated at the same time.

You can be helped, but only if you follow your physician's instructions completely.

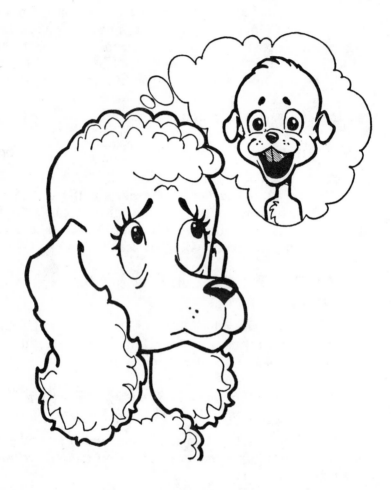

*Tetracyclines, When Taken By The Mother, May Cause Discoloration Of The Baby's Teeth.*

# 14 | Miscarriage And Labor That Starts Too Early

As we discussed earlier, a normal pregnancy is carried for 40 weeks or 280 days (counting from the first day of the last menstrual period until delivery). Normal variation is two weeks early or two weeks later than this.

However, when the baby comes earlier than this there is always some increase in risk of survival. In general, the earlier the baby comes, the less chance for survival.

## 1.  What Is A Miscarriage?

Miscarriage is loss of the baby before it weight 500 grams (1¼ pounds) or before twenty weeks of gestation. However, this definition is more legal than medical, since survival of the infant before 24 weeks is extremely rare.

## 2.  When Is An Infant Considered To Be Premature?

When it weighs between 500 grams (1¼ pounds) and 2500 grams (5½ pounds).

### 3. Why Does A Doctor Often Call A Miscarriage An Abortion, Even Though It Happened By Itself?

Intentionally performed, abortions are spoken of as "induced" abortions, as contrasted to the "spontaneous" abortions that occur by themselves. But whether spontaneous or induced, the correct medical term is abortion. The lay term is "miscarriage".

Many people falsely interpret an induced abortion to mean a "criminal" abortion. However, since the laws have been changed to legalize abortions, these are now spoken of as "therapeutic" abortions—abortions performed for the good of the mother, or in some cases, the baby.

### 4. What Is A Criminal Abortion?

This is an abortion carried out illegally and too often by someone who is not qualified to perform this type of surgery. With the change in laws legalizing abortion there is no longer any need to seek this type of abortion.

Abortion, carried out under favorable circumstances by qualified personnel is safe. Carried out under less than optimum conditions it can lead to infection, chronic illness, sterility, and occasionally death.

If abortion becomes necessary, seek competent advice, and have the procedure performed where the facilities are well-staffed and equipped.

### 5. What Causes Spontaneous Abortions?

Here are some of the common causes:
A. Abnormal eggs, abnormal sperm, or an abnormal union of these (thought to account for 25 to 50% of spontaneous abortions).
B. Abnormal conditions of the uterus.
C. Abnormalities in the afterbirth:
   a. Placenta previa (fertilized egg is implanted too

**112**

low in the uterus). This causes the afterbirth to lie ahead of the baby. If abortion does not take place, there is usually severe hemorrhage in labor and delivery.
  b. Early separation of the afterbirth (before birth of the baby).
  c. Clots in the blood vessels of the placenta, etc.
D. Abnormalities in the mother such as infections, injury, incompetent cervix (one which is unable to "contain" a pregnancy within the uterus until the proper time for delivery).
E. There are also many other causes, including hormonal imbalance, for example, which we do not fully understand.

### 6. What Are The Warning Symptoms Of Miscarriage That I Should Look For?

Bleeding and cramping are the two most common symptoms. If either of these or both become persistent and excessive; for instance:
  A. Bleeding more than a normal menstrual period.
  B. Cramping so severe that ordinary home-remedies will not stop them from intensifying. Notify your doctor immediately!

### 7. Do Bleeding And Cramps Always Mean That I Will Miscarry?

No. Nearly one third of pregnant women experience some bleeding and cramping, yet only a relatively small percent of these women actually miscarry.

### 8. Do Bleeding And Cramps Mean That The Baby Will Be Abnormal?

No. Although there is a slightly higher incidence of abnormality in those who bleed, this does not mean that

113

bleeding and cramping will always lead to an abnormal child if it fails to miscarry.

### 9. When Is A Miscarriage Beyond Hope (As Far As Saving The Baby Is Concerned)?

The pregnancy has probably passed "the point of no return" and will be sacrificed:

A. If placental (afterbirth) tissue has passed.

B. If bleeding becomes extremely heavy.

C. If the cramps become uncontrollable.

D. Or if the doctor finds the cervix is already dilating.

### 10. What Should Be Done If This Happens?

Usually, your doctor will take you to the hospital, where he can perform a D. & C. (a dilatation and curettage) or a vacutage which consists of stretching the cervix and removing the tissue involved with the pregnancy either by scraping or with suction.

In most hospitals early abortions are now performed by suction, which is often simpler as well as safer.

### 11. What About Going To Bed To Avoid Losing The Baby?

Let the doctor decide about this. Ordinarily it makes very little difference.

### 12. Does It Help To Raise My Feet And Legs When Bleeding?

No. This may only *conceal* bleeding by damming it in the vagina. It does not decrease the amount of bleeding. Nor does it prevent miscarriage.

**114**

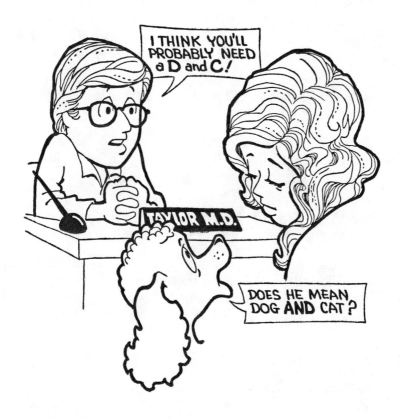

*What Should Be Done If This Happens?*

### 13. Does A Woman Always Have The Uterus Scraped Out After A Miscarriage (Have A D. & C.)?

No. Occasionally all of the products of conception (the baby and the afterbirth) are passed completely and the bleeding stops. In such a case there is no need to scrape or suction out the contents of the uterus. But your doctor must decide whether or not this is necessary.

### 14. How Do I Know That I Am Not Going Into Labor Too Early?

You may not know. However, if you begin having contractions that gradually become harder, closer together, and last longer, you may suspect early labor.

### 15. How Do I Know If The Baby Is Too Early To Survive?

This depends upon its size, vigor, and age. With improved methods of care for the premature baby, more and more are being saved at earlier ages. Few survive if more than 10 weeks early.

### 16. Does A Showing Always Mean I Will Go Into Labor?

Not always. You may or may not lose the plug of mucous from the cervix which often contains streaks of blood. This is called a "showing." Even though you have a showing and contractions, it is still possible that you may not go into true labor. Until the cervix starts to dilate, there is always a possibility of carrying your baby longer.

116

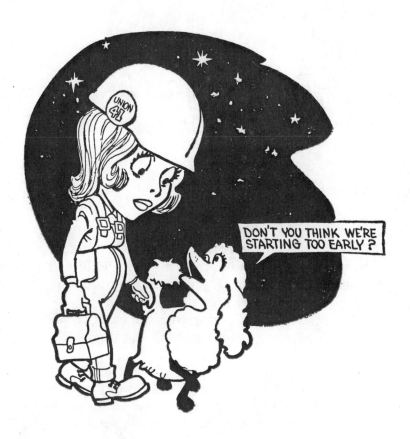

*How Do I Know That I Am Not Going Into Labor
Too Early?*

# 15 | *Bleeding Late In Pregnancy*

Bleeding early in pregnancy, before the fetus is capable of survival, often indicates miscarriage. Bleeding in the last three months of pregnancy has a different meaning. In general there are three types:

1. The SHOWING. Coming with the onset of labor, this is a plug of mucous from the cervix, often accompanied by streaks of blood. It is called the "show."

   Bleeding is slight and is followed in a few hours by labor contractions. Your doctor usually wants to know if bleeding is present, even if slight in amount.

2. PAINLESS BLEEDING. Whenever a woman has "painless bleeding" in the last three months of pregnancy, it may indicate that the afterbirth or placenta lies ahead of the baby, a condition called "placenta previa." Depending upon how much of this afterbirth lies ahead of the baby, the condition may be very serious and requires your doctor's immediate attention.

Be sure to tell your doctor how much you are bleeding, whether it is bright red blood, or dark, black blood, and also if it is accompanied by pain or not. He will then determine if immediate delivery (including cesarean operation) is necesary or if you may be allowed to wait and be watched.

3. BLEEDING ALONG WITH SEVERE ABDOMINAL PAIN. Occasionally there is bleeding "behind" the afterbirth that causes it to separate from the uterus before the baby is born. This is called "premature separation" of the placenta. If enough of the placenta is separated from the uterine wall, it can no longer deliver enough oxygen to the baby, and the baby suffocates.

Along with the pain, the mother may notice a stony hardness of her uterus, and extreme tenderness of the uterus. She should notify her doctor at once of this type of pain or bleeding.

Other questions about bleeding late in pregnancy:

1. ARE THERE OTHER CAUSES OF BLEEDING LATE IN PREGNANCY?
Yes. There may be minor causes, such as erosion of the cervix, polyps (small growths like berries), or varicose veins of the vagina that break and bleed. These can be taken care of by your doctor quite easily. However, let him make the diagnosis and decide how important the bleeding is.

2. IS IT TRUE THAT NATURAL REDHEADS AND BLONDES HAVE A TENDENCY TO BLEED MORE THAN OTHERS?
No. This is an "Old Wives Tale".

3. HOW CAN I TELL MY DOCTOR HOW MUCH I'M BLEEDING OR HOW MUCH BLOOD I HAVE LOST?
Ideally we should measure the amount. However, this is rarely practical or possible. We can report the

**119**

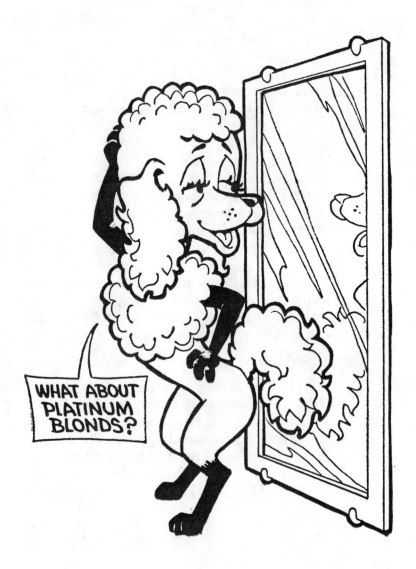

*Is It True That Natural Redheads And Blondes Have A Tendency To Bleed More Than Others?*

amount of blood in terms of thoroughly or partially soaked pads, towels, or underclothing.

Another method is to report the need for double padding, or flooding through such padding, every fifteen minutes, half-hour or such. From this information the doctor can judge whether it is an emergency or not.

If the bleeding is more than scant, he will likely want to examine you. In this event, take the soiled pads with you for examination and let him evaluate the blood loss.

# 16 | Tubal Pregnancy . . . The Displaced Person

A pregnancy anywhere besides where it should be (in the uterine cavity) is called an ectopic pregnancy. More than 90% of these ectopic pregnancies occur in the Fallopian tube. About one in every 200 pregnancies is "misplaced."

## 1. What Causes Tubal Pregnancy?

Apparently anything that delays the passage of the fertilized egg down the tube into the uterine cavity can cause this egg to be implanted in the Fallopian tube. Infection of the tube, an oversized egg, defective cilia (the small, hair-like structures lining the tubes that propel the egg on its way)—are some of the common causes.

Some studies have indicated that tubal pregnancies are conceived late in the cycle and the ensuing menstrual backwash prevents normal descent of the fertilized egg through the tube and into the uterine cavity.

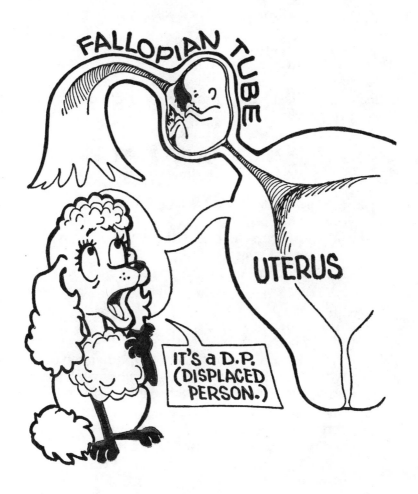

*Tubal Pregnancy...The Displaced Person*

**2.** *I Have Heard That An Intra-Uterine Device Increases The Chances Of Tubal Pregnancy. Is This True?*

We don't know exactly why, but the incidence of tubal pregnancies is about 10 times as high in women wearing an IUD. Perhaps the devices cause a low-grade infection. At least they provide no protection against tubal pregnancy.

**3.** *What Symptoms Should I Look For If I Suspect A Tubal Pregnancy?*

    a. If a menstrual period is late, prolonged, different, or even missed.

    b. If pain occurs in one side or the other with or without bleeding.

    c. Before rupture of a tubal pregnancy:

        Pain may be vague, mild, even a few cramps only.

    d. At the time of rupture:

        You may have what we call the "bathroom sign", since the sharp pain of rupture often occurs while straining with a bowel movement. Along with this severe pain, the patient may faint, or may collapse on the floor due to the pain or to the sudden loss of blood when the pregnancy ruptures through the wall of the tube.

        When rupture of the tube occurs, it often tears through some blood vessels, permitting a rapid loss of blood. Nature then drops the blood pressure (called shock) as a protective measure so that the individual does not bleed to death.

        This, of course, becomes an emergency and requires rapid diagnosis and treatment by transfusions and surgery.

### 4. Why Is A Pregnancy Test Of Little Value In Tubal Pregnancy?

It is positive in only 35% to 40% of the cases. If negative, it still does not mean that there cannot be a tubal pregnancy. When it is positive, it does not rule out a normal pregnancy in the uterus.

### 5. Why Does The Doctor Insert A Needle Into The Vagina To Make The Diagnosis of Tubal Pregnancy?

Actually the needle is inserted (via the vagina) into the lower-most part of the abdominal cavity to see if there is blood present. Non-clotting blood obtained through the needle indicates hemorrhage into the abdominal cavity, which presumably is coming from a ruptured tubal pregnancy.

### 6. Does A Tubal Pregnancy Always Require Surgery?

Almost always. Rarely the pregnancy aborts into the abdominal cavity and bleeding stops. Ordinarily it distends the Fallopian tube until it ruptures.

Bleeding usually continues until the blood vessels are occluded (clamped or tied off) at surgery. With rare exception the diagnosis of tubal pregnancy requires surgery.

### 7. If I Have Had One Tubal Pregnancy, Am I More Likely To Have Another One?

Instead of one chance in 200, your chances of getting a second one would be one in about 12.

### 8. Is There Any Chance That A Tubal Pregnancy Could Be Carried To Full Term And That A Normal Baby Could Be Delivered?

In the extremely rare cases in which this has occurred, the pregnancy became attached to the abdominal wall and continued to grow. However, such a pregnancy is hazardous because of the danger of hemorrhage even when delivered by cesarean operation (as it would have to be).

Hence, when an ectopic pregnancy of any kind is diagnosed, surgery is carried out as soon as arrangements can be completed to do so. Naturally this is not done without having started a transfusion on the patient.

126

# 17 | *What Is Toxemia Of Pregnancy?*

Toxemia is a condition found only in pregnancy, in which the blood pressure is elevated, swelling (water retention) occurs, and albumin appears in the urine. We don't know the cause, but we do know how to treat it if we discover it early.

### 1. *How Would I Know If I Had Toxemia Of Pregnancy?*

You might watch for the following signs:

A. In addition to swelling in your feet and ankles, you might notice swelling in your face, hands, and abdomen.

B. Headache is common, either in front or back.

C. Blurring of your vision. Rarely temporary blindness occurs.

D. Pain in your upper abdomen.

E. Scanty amount of urine, even when you are drinking a normal amount of water.

Any or all of these symptoms should be reported to your doctor.

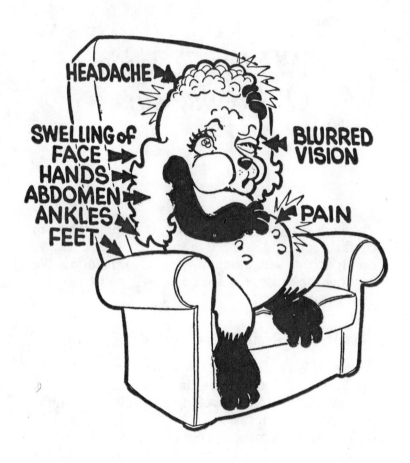

*How Would I Know If I Had Toxemia Of Pregnancy?*

## 2. But Isn't Swelling Normal For Pregnancy?

A small amount in feet and ankles is normal. Anything more than this should be reported to your doctor.

## 3. What Can I Do To Avoid Toxemia Of Pregnancy?

There is nothing we know of to avoid toxemia since we do not know the cause. However, if any of the three cardinal signs of toxemia appear (elevated blood pressure, albumin in the urine, or swelling), a woman should:

A. Force Fluids. Drink as much water as you can.
B. Get adequate sleep plus a nap if possible.
C. Report any of the above signs of toxemia to your doctor immediately!
D. Your doctor will know what to do.

## 4. What If I Don't Improve, Inspite Of These Precautions?

A. Your doctor may have to put you in the hospital where you can be observed carefully and treated actively with medicine to control your blood pressure.
B. If absolute bed rest and medicines do not control your toxemia, your baby may have to be delivered, either normally or by cesarean operation, depending upon your doctor's judgment.

## 5. What Happens If I Ignore Toxemia Of Pregnancy?

If untreated, toxemia may become worse. Convulsions, coma, and even death of the mother as well as the baby may occur. However, this is rare because most mothers are diagnosed early and adequate treatment is undertaken.

### 6. Am I Likely To Have Toxemia Again With My Next Baby?

About one third of the women who have toxemia with one baby will have it with subsequent pregnancies. Women who have repeated toxemia of pregnancy are more likely to have a permanent elevation of blood pressure following the pregnancy.

However, this does not mean that every woman who has had toxemia with one baby will have it again. Nor does it mean that she will have any after-effects following toxemia of pregnancy.

### 7. Is It Possible To Have High Blood Pressure And Not Have Toxemia Of Pregnancy?

Yes. These are two separate diseases, although they overlap somewhat. In the absence of disease, blood pressure has a tendency to become lower during pregnancy.

Women with known high blood pressure, however, would do well to have a complete study of their condition before undertaking a pregnancy.

# 18 | *You Mean More Than One!*

Generally speaking, the larger the animal and the longer it lives, the fewer offspring in its litter. Human beings are considered large and long-lived, hence the single birth pattern.

### 1. *How Common Are Twins?*

Twins occur once in 99 deliveries in the United States and once in 74 in non-whites. They are most common in blacks and least common in orientals.

### 2. *What Determines Whether They Are Identical Twins Or Not?*

When twins result from splitting of a single fertilized egg, the twins are identical. Naturally identical twins are of the same sex. However, when two separate eggs are fertilized (by two separate sperm, of course) the twins are fraternal—two brothers, two sisters, or one of each.

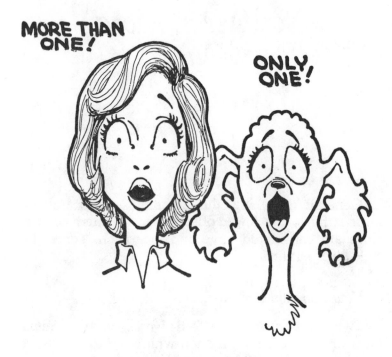

*You Mean More Than One!*

Triplets, Quadruplets, or Quintuplets may occur from various combinations of identical and fraternal twinning; or from one, two, or three eggs, etc.

### 3. Which Are More Common, Identical Or Fraternal Twins?

About 25% of twins are identical, the other 75% are fraternal.

### 4. Are Older Women More Likely To Have Twins?

Fraternal twinning increases up to age 35 to 39, but decreases after the age of 40.

Identical twinning is about the same for all ages and races.

The more children a woman has, the more likely she is to have fraternal twins.

### 5. How Can A Doctor Tell If I Am Going To Have Twins?

1. He may be able to outline them through the abdominal wall with his hands.
2. He may be able to detect two heart beats with his stethoscope.
3. Electrocardiograms of the babies' hearts will often detect twins.
4. X-rays give *positive* evidence of twins, but X-rays are not taken unless there is some definite reason for taking them, such as to detect abnormal positions.

### 6. How Often Does The Doctor "Miss" The Diagnosis Of Twins?

Correct diagnosis is made in about 70% of cases. He misses on about 30%.

133

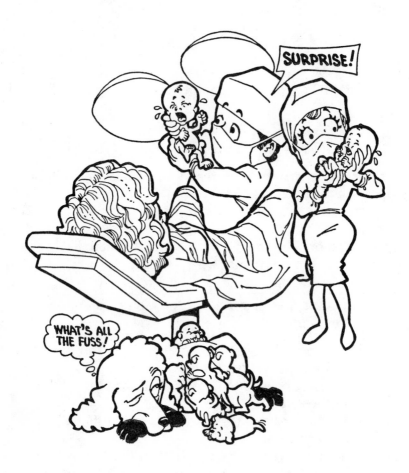

*How Often Does The Doctor "Miss" The Diagnosis Of Twins?*

### 7. How Can The Doctor Tell For Sure If The Twins Are Identical?

Usually this can be determined by examination, under the microscope, of the membranes covering the babies. Fraternal twins have completely separate membranes, whereas identical twins share part of their membranes.

### 8. Are Twin Pregnancies Likely To Have More Complications?

Yes. For instance:
1. Twins are more likely to be born prematurely, hence their chance of survival is less.
2. Mothers with twin pregnancies are more likely to have toxemia of pregnancy with its complications.
3. Varicose veins and swelling (especially in legs) are more common in mothers with twin pregnancies.
4. Defects are more common in identical twins. Twinning of this type is considered a defect—but in this case, not an undesirable one.
5. There is more false labor in twin pregnancies.
6. There is more discomfort for the mother because of the greatly distended uterus.

### 9. Is There More Hazard To Delivery Of Twin Pregnancies?

Yes—
1. There is more likely to be compression of the baby's cord due to entanglement.
2. There are more abnormal positions and therefore more problems in delivery, such as prolapse of the umbilical cord, premature separation of the afterbirth with bleeding, and more forcep (instrument) deliveries.

135

3. Hemorrhage after twin deliveries is more frequent.
4. Twin babies are smaller, usually because the mother goes into labor earlier.
5. In general, twins have less chance for survival than singletons.

## 10. Do Twins Share A Placenta Between Them?

Each twin has its own placenta, but the placentas may be located side by side so that it looks like only one oversized placenta.

## 11. How Common Are Triplets, Quadruplets, Etc.?

Assuming that twins occur approximately once in 100 deliveries, triplets occur once in 10,000 deliveries quadruplets once in 1,000,000 deliveries, etc.—.

# 19 | Xray And Your Pregnancy

When xrays are taken, a beam similar to a beam of light is passed through your body and records itself on a film, just like taking a picture. Shadows cast on this film outline bones and other structures.

Xray beams can be harmful to your child, but only if in sufficient quantity and over a sufficient length of time. Certain xrays are necessary, safe, and even life-saving during pregnancy. But unless the xrays are absolutely necessary at this time, they should be deferred until after the baby is born.

### 1. How Harmful Are Xrays Of My Teeth Or Of My Chest To My Baby?

In general, the irradiation reaching the pelvis from xrays of the chest or teeth are much less than that received from water, air, etc., in the course of a week. It is always wise to shield the abdomen when these xrays are taken, just as a precaution.

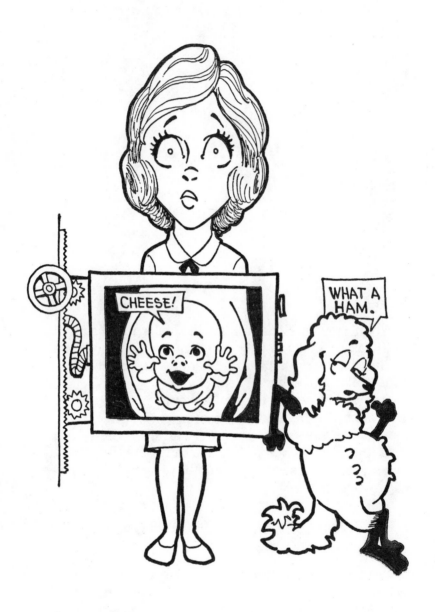

*Xray And Your Pregnancy*

## 2. When Is The Best Time To Take Xrays In Women?

If possible, these are best taken right after the menstrual period has started and before conception occurs (14 days before the onset of the next expected menstrual period, preferably no later than 10 days after the onset of a menstrual period).

## 3. Why Not Avoid Xrays Completely During Pregnancy?

Sometimes xrays are necessary—i.e. in accidents, injuries, acute urinary tract or gall bladder conditions Your doctor will weigh the benefits against the risk and decide if it is absolutely necessary during the pregnancy, or if it can wait until afterward.

## 4. Why Should Xrays Of The Chest Be Taken During Pregnancy?

If there is a good chance of tuberculosis, an xray of the chest should be taken to determine for sure. A newborn baby has no immunity against tuberculosis. To avoid exposure and possible death from tuberculosis, it is well worth while to take an xray of such a mother's chest (shielding the abdomen, of course).

## 5. Do Xrays Later In Pregnancy Also Cause Damage?

Most structures of the baby are well formed after four months. Where possible, necessary xrays should be deferred until later in the pregnancy. As stated, unnecessary xrays are avoided completely in pregnancy, regardless of the duration.

### 6.  Do Xrays Cause Cancer?

Yes, but only in doses larger than those used in properly controlled xray studies.

The use of xrays is one of the greatest boons to health in the past 50 years. Many of us owe our lives and health to xrays at some time or other in our lives. Certainly xray is safe when used properly.

# 20 | *Cesarean Births*

Once a frightening and dangerous experience, cesarean birth (delivery through an abdominal incision) is now one of the safest major operations. Even with the many serious conditions for which cesarean may be performed, the mortality is only 1 in 400 operations.

About one in every 18 or 20 deliveries is a cesarean, although some hospitals may show an incidence many times higher.

### 1. Is It True That "Once A Cesarean, Always A Cesarean?"

If the same reason is still present (too small pelvis, for instance), then the operation will have to be repeated with each succeeding pregnancy. If this indication is no longer present, then it is left to the judgment of the doctor about performing another cesarean operation or allowing normal delivery through the vagina.

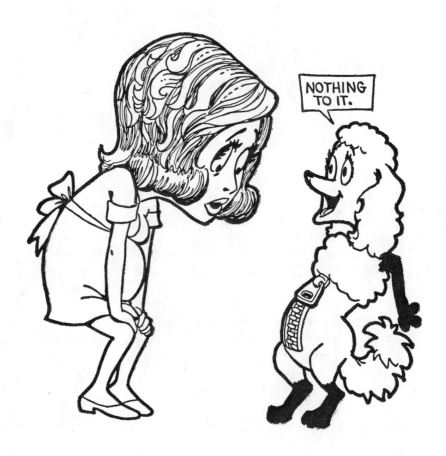

*Cesarean Births*

## 2. What Is The Commonest Cause Of Cesarean Birth?

A "previous" cesarean birth. Depending upon the method used for the first cesarean operation, your doctor decides whether to allow labor and delivery through the vagina. Other causes of cesarean may be a narrow pelvis, a large infant, unsatisfactory progress in labor, toxemia, placenta previa, prolapsed umbilical cord, etc.

## 3. Is There A Greater Risk To The Baby By Cesarean?

Yes—BUT—this depends upon the reason for the cesarean. A higher fetal mortality rate, for example, may be due to prematurity of the infant, placenta previa (afterbirth ahead of the baby) with the accompanying hemorrhage, or many other causes.

## 4. Is Cesarean Operation Ever Performed After Death Of The Mother—To Save The Infant?

Yes. In fact, failure to try to save the infant in event of death of a pregnant woman is considered negligence from a medical and legal point of view.

## 5. How Many Babies Can A Woman Have By Cesarean?

There is actually no set limit. However, much depends upon the condition of the uterus, how it has healed, the general condition of the mother, etc.

## 6. Can A Woman Who Has A Cesarean Operation Nurse Her Baby?

Yes, and many of them do.

7. *Can A Woman Be Sterilized At The Same Time She Has A Cesarean Operation?*

Yes. The Fallopian tubes are in perfect view and can be "tied" at the time of the surgery.

8. *Can The Uterus Be Removed (Hysterectomy) At The Time A Cesarean Operation Is Performed?*

Yes. This is necessary in certain cases. The operation carries a slightly higher risk than cesarean alone, but it is very successful.

# 21 | *Weight And See*

A most significant change, in fact a complete about-face has taken place in our attitude toward diet and pregnancy. Only a few years ago doctors placed the greatest emphasis on limitation of weight in pregnancy, primarily to avoid toxemia of pregnancy. In the past few years, however, we have become more aware of the importance of adequate nutrition for the mother and fetus.

Failure to meet the nutritional needs of pregnancy may have some far-reaching effects upon the unborn child. Let's discuss a few questions covering this subject.

**1.** *Is Excessive Weight Gain During Pregnancy Really Harmful To The Mother Or The Baby?*

Yes. It is still important not to gain too much weight, since the mother may have a greater tendency to develop complications of pregnancy. Nor does it help her morale to pile on those unnecessary, plaguing pounds of weight.

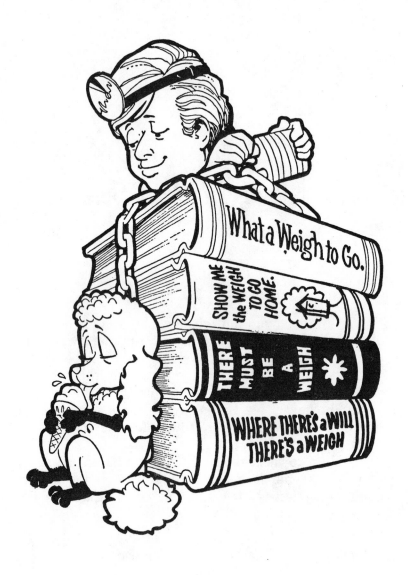

*Weight And See*

Also, there is a definite relationship between the weight gain of the mother and that of the baby. This means that she could have a more difficult delivery because of the increased size of the baby.

## 2. What Is Considered "Excessive" Weight Gain?

We might better ask, "What is normal weight gain in pregnancy?" This may vary with each patient, depending upon whether she is overweight to begin with, her general health, body build and stature, etc. . . .

In general the average woman's weight gain in pregnancy is distributed as follows:

| | |
|---|---|
| Weight of baby | 7 pounds |
| Weight of afterbirth | 1 pound |
| Weight of amniotic fluid | 2 pounds |
| Increased weight of uterus | 2 pounds |
| Increased weight of breasts | 2 pounds |
| Excess water & fat in preg. | 6 pounds |

Total—20 pounds

Thus you see, an average weight gain of 18 to 24 pounds is about ideal. However, some overweight women may gain no weight while an underweight woman may happily gain 30 pounds or even more.

The optimum weight for you will be determined by your doctor.

## 3. Can I Obtain Sufficient Vitamins From The Foods I Eat—The Natural Way?

Indeed you can and you should. Because most of our modern foods are "fortified" with vitamins, this presents no problem.

However, there are some cases in which the doctor may feel additional vitamins are needed.

### 4. What Should A Pregnant Woman Have In Her Diet?

There are three basic groups of essential foods:
1. Proteins—for growth and repair of your body.
2. Minerals and vitamins—for growth and to keep your body in good working condition.
3. Fats and carbohydrates—for energy.

A good diet contains a balance of these. Some women consult charts, but by far most pregnant women want a simple rule of thumb to direct them in preparation of healthy meals.

### 5. What Are The Basic Food Groups?

There are six:
1. Milk group.
2. Meat group
3. Vegetable group
4. Bread and cereal group
5. Fats and oils
6. Sugars and sweets

### 6. What Is The Danger In Food Fads—Vegetarian Or Fruitarian Diets, For Instance?

Although it is possible to obtain adequate protein in these diets, it is difficult and requires more knowledge and care than most people have about nutrition. On such a diet it is also difficult to obtain sufficient protein without boredom.

### 7. What Is An Adequate Amount Of Protein For Pregnancy?

The Protein Requirements of Pregnancy are:

| Food | Regular | Lacto-Ovo Vegetarian | Lacto Veg. | Pure Veg. |
|---|---|---|---|---|
| 1½ pints milk | 27 | 27 | 27 | — |
| 2 servings meat (6 oz.) | 36 | — | — | — |
| 2 eggs | | —12 | — | — |
| ½ cup cottage cheese | — | 22 | 22 | — |
| 4 tablespoons peanut butter | — | — | 17 | 17 |
| 2 cups lentils, pinto beans | — | — | — | 36 |
| 3 servings vegetables | 6 | 6 | 6 | 6 |
| 3 slices bread | 6 | 6 | 6 | 6 |
| 4 servings fruits | 2 | 2 | 2 | 2 |
| Total— | 77 | 78 | 80 | 67 |

## 8. Are There Certain Women Who Need Special Attention To Their Diet Needs In Pregnancy?

Yes. The following groups may especially require help:

1. Women under 17 years of age. These women are still growing and maturing in addition to meeting the needs of pregnancy.
2. Women who have babies very close together may deplete normal reserves.
3. Women who are underweight before starting a pregnancy have a double demand.
4. Women who are overweight. Often because their eating habits are faulty and consist of sweets, carbohydrates, etc., they are found to be protein-deficient.
5. Food-faddists may have considerably more difficulty in meeting the needs of their pregnancies.

6. Low-income mothers may be saving on food to meet other needs.

### 9. Is It Wrong, Then, For Me To Try To Lose Weight During Pregnancy?

There may be exceptions, but there is usually too much danger of compromising the nutrition of the developing infant when a mother tries to decrease her calories sufficiently to lose weight. This weight loss is better accomplished AFTER the birth of the baby.

### 10. Could You Give Me Hints To Cut Down On My Calorie Intake?

Here are a few suggestions that may help:
1. Take a good inventory of your habits.
2. Choose a sensible diet pattern with realistic exercise periods.
3. You may want to change your eating habits by shifting from the normal three meals to five or six small meals a day.
4. When possible, serve and eat meals buffet-style rather than family style—this eliminates the temptation for having second and third helpings.
5. Use a smaller plate and cut your food into smaller pieces.
6. Break the "clean plate" habit.
7. Take a long "meal break." Most people eat much less if they take time to eat slowly.
8. For an added incentive paste pictures of slim women on your cupboard or refrigerator doors.
9. Drink water! It is assimilated quickly, aiding digestion and elimination. It is also filling. Drink plenty of water, especially upon arising and between meals. And it contains NO calories!
10. Never eat when over-tired or upset. Make an effort to relax before eating. Tension can undo many of the benefits of a well-balanced meal.

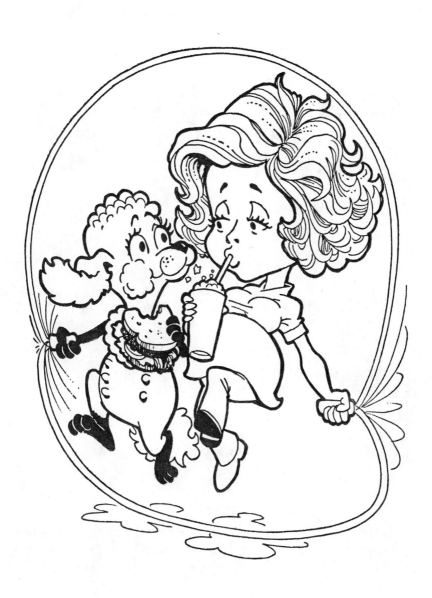

*Could You Give Me Hints To Cut Down On My Calorie Intake?*

# 22 | How Do I Know When To Go And What To Do?

There is one thing sure about pregnancy—it cannot go on forever. If you are pregnant, you know that some time you will have to start labor.

The big question with the first pregnancy is "Doctor, how will I know when I am really in labor?" Generally speaking, it's like being in love, if you have to ask someone if you are then you aren't.

### 1. Will I Know When My Baby "Drops?"

Several weeks prior to the onset of labor, the baby usually "drops" or "settles" downward. You may, or may not, be aware of this.

This change is the result of the baby's head descending into the pelvic cavity. The baby simply drops into a more favorable position for birth.

### 2. Will I Feel Better Or Worse With This Change?

You could experience both. Upper abdominal pressure is usually relieved when this occurs causing the mother's breathing to be easier.

You may, however, experience a more frequent desire to empty your bladder due to increased pressure upon your bladder. You may also have cramp-like pains in your thighs, and walking could be a bit more difficult.

### 3. What Are "Braxton-Hicks Contractions?"

During pregnancy it is normal for the muscles of the uterus to intermittently tighten. The uterus becomes almost stony hard, then relaxes and becomes soft again. These tightenings are known as "Braxton-Hicks" contractions, and because they are mild, they often go unnoticed.

As the estimated date of confinement approaches, however, these contractions become cramp-like and uncomfortable. These "Braxton-Hicks" contractions are sometimes confused with true labor. Actually this is just one of nature's ways of preparing for true labor.

### 4. What Is False Labor?

For a varying period before true labor is established, pregnant women often experience and are sometimes confused by so-called "false labor". Unlike true labor, false labor pains usually occur at irregular intervals and they are confined chiefly to the lower part of the abdomen and groin.

The duration of false labor contractions is usually short—30 seconds or less—and unlike true labor contractions, they are rarely intensified by walking. On the contrary, they may be relieved by moving about or just resting.

Instead of increasing in intensity, duration and frequency, false labor contractions diminish and finally disappear altogether. There may be several episodes of false labor extending over many days before true labor actually starts.

False labor, however, is much less common in "first" pregnancies.

## 5. How Will I Know When I Am Actually In Labor?

True labor usually begins with an intermittent backache, or a feeling of discomfort in your abdomen similar to menstrual cramps. As your uterus contracts, your abdomen becomes stony hard, then as the contraction ends, your abdomen feels soft again.

True labor contractions may be spaced at regular intervals, 8 to 20 minutes apart, and lasting over 30 seconds. It is important that you time your contractions both as to the interval between them and their duration. One reason they are called "labor contractions" and not "labor pains," is that they are not always painful.

If you feel intermittent backache or a tightening of your abdomen, place your hands over your abdomen and start timing. From the time the abdomen becomes stony hard until the time it again becomes soft, is the duration. From the time the abdomen becomes hard until the time it becomes hard again, is the interval between contractions.

Do not guess at the timing! You must be able to give accurate information to your doctor when you call him. When your contractions become regular at five to eight minute intervals and last from 20 to 30 seconds, you should leave for the hospital.

Take into consideration how far you live from the hospital, how long it takes you to get there, and how uncomfortable you are. If you are not able to relax between contractions, you should go to the hospital regardless of whether they are regular or not! It might be a good idea to make a "dry run" to the hospital to determine the best route and your driving time.

154

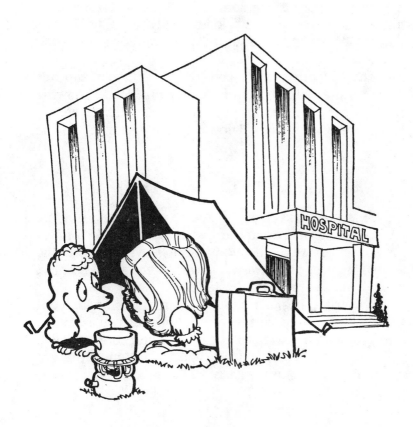

*How Will I Know When I Am Actually In Labor?*

### 6. Does a "Bloody-Show" Always Mean That I Am In Labor?

Not always. When your doctor performs a pelvic examination during the last month of pregnancy for instance, it may cause some bleeding for the next few hours. However, a true "bloody show" usually appears when contractions have started or when they are about to start.

The "bloody show" consists of a plug of mucous containing a few streaks of blood. This bloody showing should not be confused with *active* bleeding. If the bleeding looks more like menstrual flow call your doctor, it could be important.

### 7. When Will My "Bag Of Waters" Break?

This may take place days—or even weeks—before labor starts. It may occur during labor, or your doctor may "break" it before the delivery of the baby. Whenever the waters break spontaneously, however, you should contact your doctor or go to the hospital.

If you are near term when your waters break, your labor will probably start within 24 hours. If you are not at term, then your doctor will decide the best course for you to follow. He will probably give you precautions to prevent infection if he allows you to go home to continue your pregnancy.

### 8. When Should I Notify My Doctor That I Am In Labor?

Some doctors prefer to know immediately when your contractions begin. Many prefer to be notified when true labor can be identified (as noted above). Others prefer that you go directly to the hospital, and let the labor and delivery personnel contact him.

Your doctor will probably advise you well in advance

156

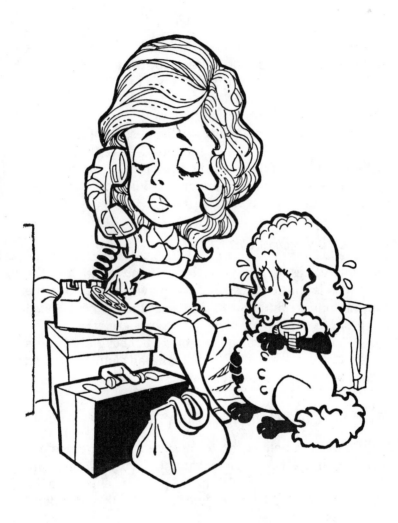

*When Should I Notify My Doctor That I Am In Labor?*

as to his preference. If he overlooks doing this, remember to ask him on one of your visits.

### 9. What Do They Mean By "Dilated?"

This refers to the cervix or neck of the uterus. As the uterus becomes tense and contracted, the force is referred to the cervix, where it causes the cervix to thin out, stretch, and gradually open. The amount of opening is then referred to as dilatation.

As the cervix dilates to allow the presenting part of the baby to pass through, it is measured in centimeters or inches. Full dilatation (wide open) is a diameter of approximately 10 centimeters or 4 to 5 inches, which will permit the baby to be born.

### 10. How Long Does Labor Last?

This varies according to the size and position of the baby in relation to the size of the pelvis, how strong the contractions are and how many babies the mother has had (each succeeding labor usually becomes easier).

Averages do not mean too much, but beyond 24 hours for the first stage is considered abnormally long. Less than 3 hours labor is unusually short.

### 11. What Can I Do To Help Labor?

Relaxation helps labor to progress. Some women can relax during labor, others cannot. Many women are relaxed when they arrive at the hospital and check into the labor unit. In fact, some become so relaxed they wonder if their labor has subsided.

Since labor contractions are involuntary, they are more effective if they are not interfered with. Fear renders them less effective, and anxiety often prolongs labor.

During the first part of your labor, it is best that you

158

relax as much as possible. Take deep breaths as contractions occur and rest between contractions. To help accomplish this, try to "unwrinkle" your forehead and allow your facial muscles to sag. This often aids in relaxing other parts of your body. Many women find it helpful to exhale a little more than they inhale.

If you tighten your hands you are less likely to relax. Place your hands over your abdomen or allow them to hang loosely at your side. Contrary to common practice, try not to "grip" your husband's hand.

### 12. What Does It Mean When Someone Mentions Different "Stages Of Labor?"

Labor is the process whereby the baby and afterbirth are expelled from the body. In labor there are three stages:

First Stage—Begins when your cervix begins to open up or dilate. Ends when your cervix is fully opened or dilated.

Second Stage—Begins when your cervix is fully dilated and ends when your baby is is delivered.

Third Stage—Begins as soon as your baby is delivered and ends when your afterbirth is delivered.

### 13. Will Drugs To Relieve Pain Harm My Baby?

If drugs are given only as your doctor recommends, they are safe. However, do not insist upon more medicine than you actually need. Too often pain pills are requested when you are merely anxious and upset, rather than in pain.

Remember that a certain amount of nearly every drug is passed through your afterbirth into your baby. Although your doctor wants to relieve your discomfort, both you and your doctor want to insure the safe deliverance of your baby.

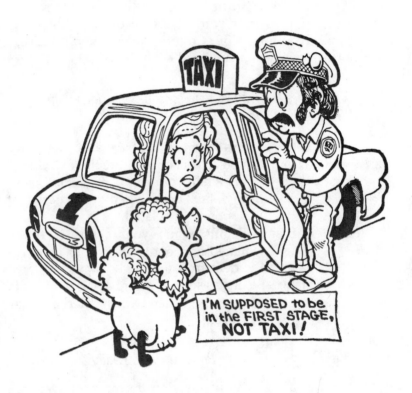

What Does It Mean When Someone Mentions Different
"Stages Of Labor?"

## 14. Does It Help To Push With Labor Contractions?

Not in the first stage. When your cervix is not fully dilated, pushing has a tendency to stretch your bladder, rectum and pelvic floor unnecessarily, without helping to dilate your cervix.

Pushing before you are told to, may cause these organs to sag and lose their support after the pregnancy is over.

## 15. Will I Be Able To Eat During Labor?

Food does not digest well during labor and tends to "lie" uncomfortably in the stomach. It is best to take only small amounts of clear liquids or a few ice chips.

If there is a possibility that you would be having a general anesthetic, your doctor will probably ask you not to take anything by mouth after you start labor.

161

# 23 | Delivery—So This Is How It Is!

Delivery of the baby is another name for the *second stage* of labor. It is the process of actual birth of your baby through the vagina and consists of some twisting, turning, moulding, and expelling of your baby.

### 1. How Do I Know When My Cervix Is Fully Dilated (Open)?

At this time you will actually have an uncontrollable urge to bear down and to expel your baby. If you have had a spinal anesthetic, you may not have this urge. However, your doctor can tell you when you have reached this stage and he will direct you to "bear down" with your labor pains.

### 2. How Does My Baby Actually Come Out?

Your baby usually delivers head-first with its "crown" making the first appearance. Next comes the forehead, with the brow, eyes, nose, mouth, and chin appearing in succession. The baby "looks" down at the floor.

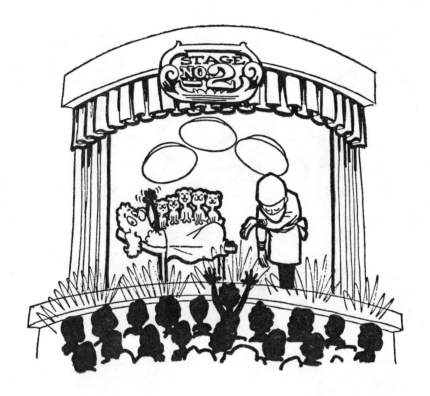

*Delivery—So This Is How It Is!*

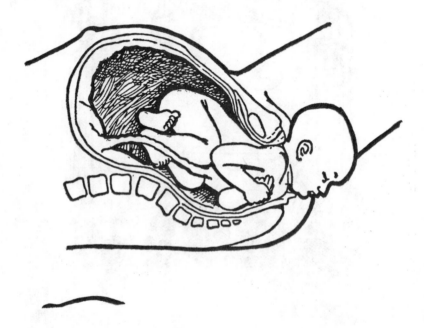

*How Does My Baby Actually Come Out?*

The head then rotates to either side and the shoulders appear one at a time and are delivered. The rest of the baby's body follows the shoulders without any difficulty.

### 3. Does The Baby Have To Be Spanked To Make It Breathe?

No. This is an old wives tale. Most babies breathe on their own as soon as the mucous is wiped from their mouths and throats.

If a baby fails to breathe spontaneously the doctor will gently rub its back—this causes it to gasp and take its first breath.

### 4. What Happens To All The Water That Is Normally Around The Baby?

If it has not slowly leaked out during labor and delivery it gushes from the uterus when the bag of water breaks or while the baby is being born.

### 5. What Is The Danger Of A Dry Birth If The Bag of Waters Breaks And All The Water Leaks Out?

If the bag of water breaks several days or weeks before delivery, (and labor does not ensue), more water is formed. If it occurs just before delivery, there is still sufficient water for lubrication. A so-called "dry birth" is practically non-existent.

### 6. Does It Help For Me To Push Or Bear Down During Delivery?

Yes. In the second stage with the cervix fully open you will feel as though you have to push. However, try to push only when your doctor tells you to do so.

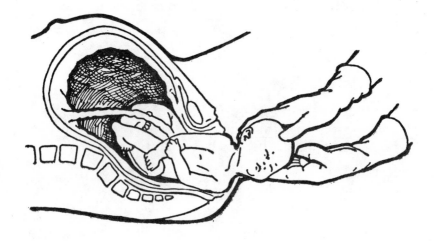

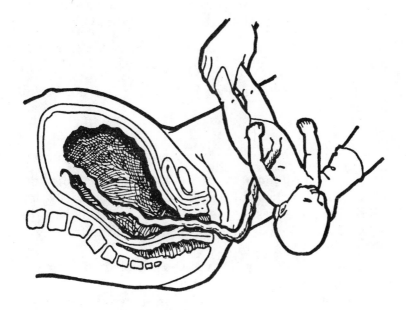

### 7. What Happens To My Large Uterus After My Baby Is Born?

Since the uterus is made up of interlacing circular bands of muscle fibers, these fibers simply contract and squeeze down around the blood vessels so that hemorrhage does not occur.

The uterus is an adaptable organ that enlarges to accommodate a growing pregnancy, and then decreases in size as your baby and afterbirth are delivered.

### 8. Should I Massage The Uterus To Help It Contract?

No. If such a manuever is necessary your doctor will take care of it.

### 9. What Is An Episiotomy?

This is a cut made by the doctor at the opening of the vagina to allow the baby to come through more easily. If it is not made, the tissues must stretch to accommodate the baby's head. If the tissue is unable to stretch sufficiently, it may tear into the rectum, etc.

An episiotomy also saves considerable pushing and straining on the part of the mother. It may also save injury to your child due to prolonged pressure of your baby's head against rigid tissues.

An episiotomy wound is also easier for the doctor to repair and it may heal better than a jagged tear. The extent of an episiotomy is more easily controlled and thus prevents a tear into your rectum.

### 10. But—Isn't It Better To Let Nature Take Care Of This Problem? After All, A Woman Is Made To Have Babies. Can't I Stretch That Much Without Tearing?

Possibly. But then again, you might *not* stretch

**168**

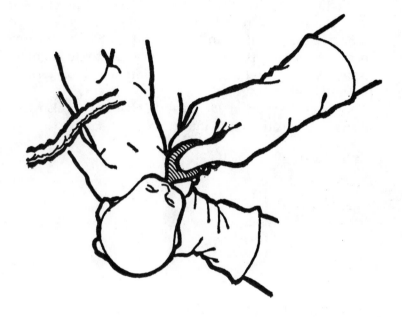

without tearing. It is also likely that your tissues may be overstretched so that they do not return to normal. This leaves the supporting structures loose and saggy in the floor of your pelvis.

Sometimes the skin does not appear torn, but your deeper tissues are torn and they fail to heal together as they should. This leaves a poorly supported pelvic "floor."

When this occurs, you may later have difficulty with your bladder and rectum, or just a distressing feeling of "things falling out." An episiotomy not only prevents these complications but it also allows a doctor to "tighten" tissues that may have been overstretched or torn by previous deliveries.

A well-supported vagina and pelvic floor is also more desirable for satisfactory intercourse.

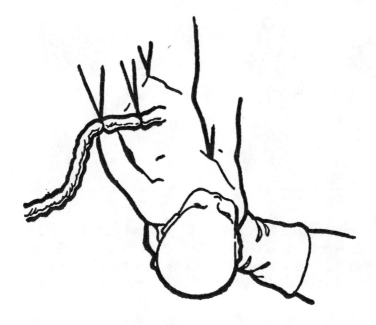

# 24 | Afterbirths . . . You Mean There's More?

Unless it has been explained beforehand, a woman may be surprised to find that she is not through with the "production" even though her baby has been delivered. There is still the matter of the placenta, or afterbirth, which must be delivered.

Usually this comes away spontaneously within twenty minutes or less after delivery of the baby. Rarely is it accompanied by more than a few cramps and moderate bleeding. Delivery of the placenta is called the THIRD STAGE of labor.

## 1. When Is Bleeding After Delivery Considered Abnormal?

More than a pint of blood loss is considered excessive whether it appears rapidly or slowly over the next 24 hours. Sometimes a little blood covers a lot of area and appears to be a hemorrhage when it is not.

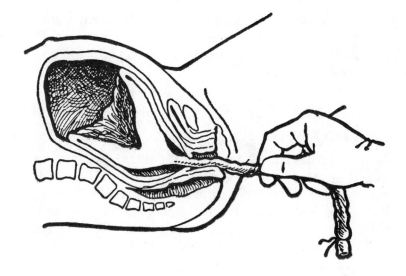

*Afterbirths...You Mean There's More?*

173

**2. Is There Anything I Should Look For Myself During This Stage Of Labor?**

Your doctor and nurse will be watching you carefully, but if there is a question in your mind, or if you think you are bleeding too much, be sure to call their attention to it.

**3. Will It Help To Stop The Bleeding If I Raise My Feet Or If You Raise The Foot Of My Bed?**

No. It might conceal the bleeding for awhile, but it simply allows the blood to accumulate in your vagina. The blood may then come out in a gush when you stand up or go to the bathroom.

**4. What Causes Bleeding After The Baby Is Born?**

ATONY: One common cause of bleeding after delivery of the baby is failure of the uterus to contract so that the open blood vessels are shut off. This is called atony, or loss of tone in the muscular walls of the uterus. If the uterus remains boggy, the blood vessels that supplied blood to the afterbirth (during pregnancy) remain open and continue to pour out blood.

Massage of the uterus along with certain drugs that make the uterus contract soon stop this type of bleeding.

TEARS OR LACERATIONS: Another cause of bleeding is found in small or large tears that have escaped attention. These may be in the uterus, the cervix, or the vagina. Examination by your doctor soon uncovers such bleeding, and a few well-placed stitches bring such bleeding rapidly under control.

RETAINED PIECES OF AFTERBIRTH: Another cause of bleeding is incomplete delivery of the placenta. If a part of the afterbirth is left in the uterus, bleeding usually continues until it is removed.

Immediately after delivery of the placenta, the doctor examines it to make certain no piece of it is missing. This is

**174**

similar to examining a pie to make sure that no piece has been cut from it. If the doctor determines that part of the placenta is not there, or if he suspects that there might be placental tissue remaining in the uterus, he will examine the uterus with his gloved hand and remove the fragment.

Only in rare instances is it necessary to use an instrument to remove the tissue. Occasionally bleeding occurs after you have been taken back to your room, or even after you have gone home from the hospital. Any bleeding that you feel is excessive should be reported to your doctor or the nurse immediately.

### 5. Is There Anything I Can Do To Prevent Hemorrhage?

No. Sometimes a very rapid or a very difficult labor will cause the uterus to fail to contract (atony). A very large baby, a small pelvis, tissues that do not "give," or a very rapid delivery sometimes will cause tears. But your doctor will exercise skill in avoiding such tears, even when instruments are necessary. However, sometimes such complications are unavoidable.

Rarely there are clotting defects in your blood and these must be corrected by your doctor. Your doctor has ways of testing for these defects and can usually correct them without difficulty.

In general, the best thing you can do is to cooperate fully with your nurses and doctor. You may be sure they will do all they can to make your delivery as comfortable, safe, and satisfying as possible.

# 25 | *About Nursing . . .*

1. *Do Babies Get Along Just As Well On Formula As They Do With Breast Feeding?*

   There are many advantages to breast feeding a baby:
   A. It establishes a closer, more intimate relationship between mother and child. Babies need to be coddled.
   B. Nursing seems to help the uterus return to normal size and function faster. Bleeding is often less, and the involution (decrease in size) is more complete in nursing mothers.
   C. Mothers need to take time out to sit down or lie down long enough to nurse their babies.
   D. There is some evidence to suggest that mothers who nurse their babies have a lower incidence of cancer of the breast.
   E. Many allergies are avoided when a mother nurses her baby. Sensitivity to certain milk products is avoided.
   F  Babies who nurse are less "sour" when spitting up.

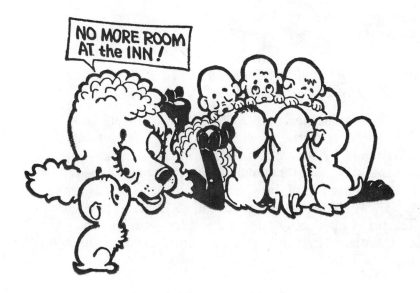

*Do Babies Get Along Just As Well On Formula*
*As They Do With Breast Feeding?*

G. Your own breast milk is the one thing no one else can give your baby.

## 2. But Won't Nursing Make Me Lose My Figure?

This is a misconception. Support or loss of support (and size) in breasts is more often due to heredity and weight loss or gain. In general, there is no proof that nursing causes mothers to lose the contour, size, or consistency of breasts more than if they did not nurse.

## 3. Is There Anything I Should Do To Prepare To Nurse My Baby?

The commonest problem is not the lack of milk supply. It is soreness of the nipples. Sometimes nipples can be toughened by soaking them in concentrated salt-water, but this may make them more irritated in some women.

Rubbing the nipples with a dry wash-cloth or towel each day helps to toughen them. Others have used Tincture of Benzoin with good results. Avoid lotions and ointments, since these seem to soften, rather than toughen nipples.

Daily massage of breasts, especially if there is fluid (called colostrum) coming from the nipples. The breast should be gently massaged to express this secretion from the nipple as follows:

Begin well above the breast and massage toward the areola (pigmented area surrounding the nipple).

Repeat movement, beginning underneath the breast and lifting the breast as you massage.

178

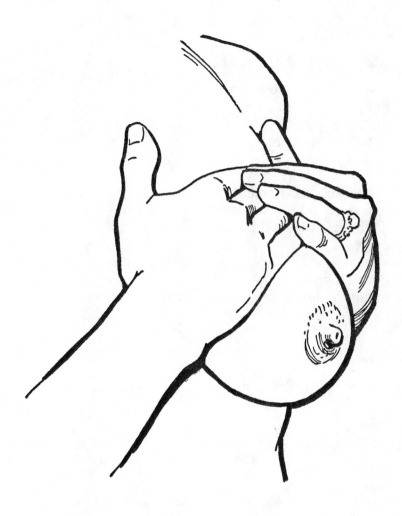

*Begin well above the breast and massage toward the areola (pigmented area surrounding the nipple).*

Using both hands on sides of breast massage toward the areola.
Repeat these exercises 10 times morning and night.

NIPPLE ROLLING EXERCISE:

Use thumb and forefinger in rolling motion on nipple to improve its erectibility. Repeat 10 times morning and night.

Use thumb and forefinger to express colostrum each day. This keeps milk ducts open.

Position infant's mouth on breast properly for most efficient nursing.

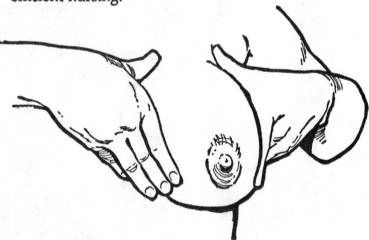

*Repeat movement, beginning underneath the breast and lifting the breast as you massage.*

180

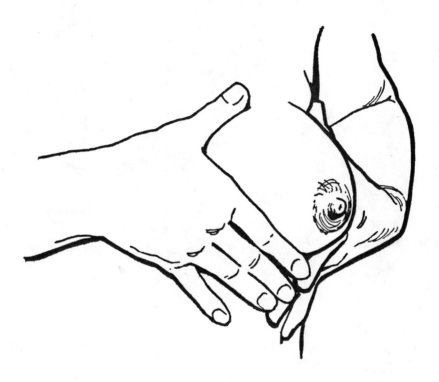

*Using both hands on sides of breast massage toward the areola.*
*Repeat these exercises 10 times morning and night.*

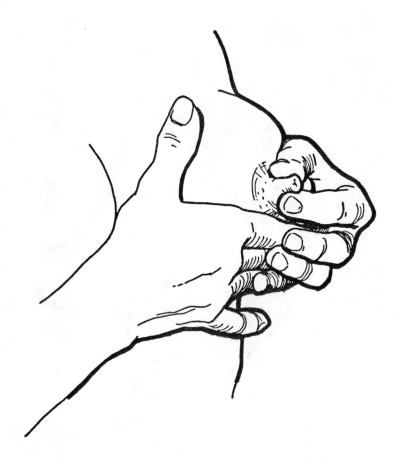

*Use thumb and forefinger in rolling motion on nipple to improve its erectibility. Repeat 10 times morning and night.*

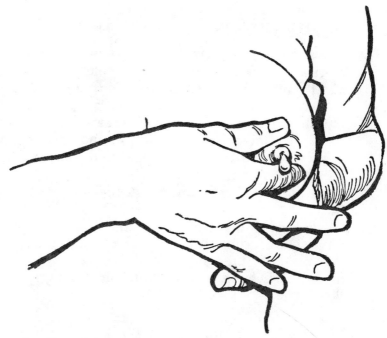

*Use thumb and forefinger to express colostrum each day.*
*This keeps milk ducts open.*

### Is There Any Way To Prevent Sagging Of The Breasts After Pregnancy?

As mentioned, this is most often due to hereditary lack of support. However, much of this sagging can be overcome by correct posture and a proper brassiere.

A well-fitting brassiere is one that has a broad nonslip strap (padded, if necessary) over the shoulders and a broad belt-type support underneath the cup.

Before the final selection of the brassiere, a woman will want to make sure the straps stay in place, and that the cups cover the entire breast when she raises her arms. If a mother intends to nurse, she should buy a nursing bra to wear during her pregnancy, since this will allow for the increasing size of her breasts.

183

## 5. How Do I Start To Nurse My Baby?

A nurse will show you how to hold the baby and to place the nipple in his mouth. Fortunately he already has a sucking reflex that tells him what to do from this point.

Although it is permissible to place the baby at the breast before the milk comes in, be sure you do not allow him to suck more than a minute at the most, or his chewing reflex will make the nipple sore. Nothing seems to stop the milk quicker than sore nipples.

Allow the baby to get a good hold on the nipple (including the dark area around the nipple); otherwise he will not be able to get much milk and he will just irritate the nipple. When you want him to discontinue nursing, break the suction by pressing some of the breast away from his mouth. To avoid pain, do not pull him forcibly away from the nipple.

## 6. How Shall I Take Care Of The Nipple?

Simple washing before and after the nursing is adequate. Do not use alcohol or other detergents. Mild soap is permitted, but be sure to rinse thoroughly before nursing.

If nipples become sore, use Tincture of Benzoin, or one of the many anesthetic ointments available. Also, by nursing completely on one side only, there will be more time for the unused nipple to heal itself. Leaving the nipple exposed to the air (by wearing a loose fitting gown) may also help to heal it along with a heat-lamp treatment.

## 7. How Long Should I Nurse My Baby?

Other foods are added as early as one month, depending upon your doctor, and as early as four months you may be able to start your baby drinking from a cup. This will eliminate bottle feeding entirely except for water in the earlier months.

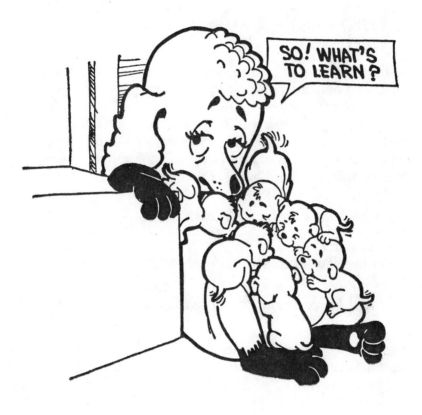

*How Do I Start To Nurse My Baby?*

### 8. What If I Have Very Small Breasts?

The size of the breasts usually has little to do with a woman's ability to nurse. If you want to nurse, you should try.

### 9. What If I Just Don't Have Quite Enough Milk For My Baby?

The amount of mother's milk will usually change to meet the demands of the baby. However, if your supply does not satisfy your baby, he will also do well on formula.

Although breast feeding is desirable, it is better to have a happy, satisfied baby (and mother) than to struggle to nurse your baby on an inadequate milk supply or with breast milk that does not agree with your baby.

### 10. Can A Mother Nurse Twins?

Yes, in most cases the supply will usually increase to meet the demand of two.

### 11. Will I Become Fat If I Nurse My Baby?

No—unless you eat too much. It is not necessary to "eat for two" when nursing. A regular diet with plenty of liquids, even water, will ordinarily produce sufficient milk for your baby.

### 12. Must I Be Careful What I Eat If I Nurse My Baby?

Many (most) medicines are carried into the milk. Nicotine from smoking, alcohol, and also laxatives find their way into the milk. These should be avoided, or at least kept to a minimum.

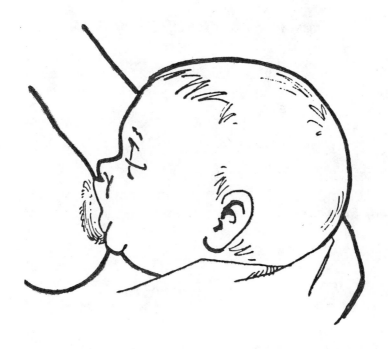

*Position infant's mouth on breast properly for most efficient nursing.*

187

**13. How Do I Know If My Baby Is Getting Enough To Eat When I Nurse?**

The baby will let you know in most cases. Otherwise, the scales will certainly tell the story.

**14. If I Deliver By Cesarean Operation, Can I Still Nurse My Baby?**

Yes. You may get off to a slower start, because you don't have close contact for approximately two days, but there is no reason why you cannot nurse if you desire to.

**15. If I Decide Not To Nurse, How Can I Prevent The Milk From Coming In?**

Your doctor can give you pills or a shot to prevent the milk from coming in. If the milk does come in, the shot or the pills will ease the discomfort enough that it can be tolerated.

**16. Are There Other Ways Of Relieving The Pain Associated With "Drying Up" The Breasts?**

Yes. Ice packs help. Binding the breasts helps somewhat. A tight bra is helpful but not sufficient.

To stop the flow of milk or to stop the discomfort, use a series of elastic bandages six to eight inches in width as wrap-arounds over your chest and breasts. It is better to completely empty the breasts before applying these bands.

Once you decide not to nurse, have the baby empty the breast completely. Then, do not nurse again, even to relieve the discomfort, or you will have to start over each time with the drying-up process.

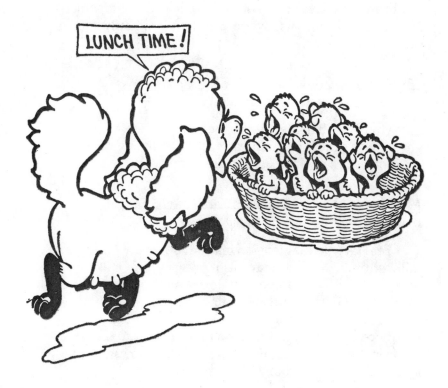

*How Do I Know If My Baby Is Getting Enough
To Eat When I Nurse?*

### 17. How Can I Tell The Difference Between Infection And Plain Engorgement Of My Breasts?

Engorgement does not cause fever, nor does it cause redness. The pain of engorgement is general throughout the breast, whereas the pain of infection is usually localized and points toward one spot. Engorgement involves both breasts, while infection ordinarily affects only one breast.

### 18. Are Mothers Who Nurse Their Babies Less Likely To Develop Cancer?

This is debatable. Some medical studies have suggested less cancer of the breasts among nursing mothers. At least it does not increase the risk of cancer of the breast.

### 19. Should I Nurse My Baby Even Though I Have A Tendency To Become Nervous?

Yes. Its true that tension may cut down on a mother's milk supply, and it may also prevent the milk from "coming in." It is important to learn to relax and get comfortable before nursing your baby.

But most women find breast feeding exerts a calming influence upon them. It forces a busy mother to take time out from her other responsibilities. The mother can coddle, love, and enjoy her baby while she nurses it.

### 20. Does Nursing A Baby "Drain" A Woman Of Her Energy?

No. Many people think it does, but all new mothers get tired whether they are nursing their babies or not. Possibly the mother who must make formula, sterilize bottles and warm the milk gets a little more tired than the mother who simply cuddles her baby to her breast while she nurses him. There may be exceptions to this rule, however.

### 21. Does Breast Feeding Save Money?

Yes. The mother who breast feeds could save enough money, which would ordinarily be spent on formula, bottles, etc., to buy a major household appliance or hire household help during the period she is nursing.

### 22. If I Nurse—Can I Be Away From My Baby For A Few Hours Or Days?

Yes. You may pump the milk and freeze it for the baby while you are away, or use a formula. Then, while you are away, pump your breast several times a day to keep comfortable and to maintain the milk supply. Separation is not easy for the baby, because he needs his mother—not just her milk.

To travel with a breastfed baby is much easier than with one on formula. Your baby can become very portable when you breastfeed him.

### 23. If I Have A Premature Baby Can I Nurse Him Just The Same?

Yes. The same procedure could be used as above, the milk being sent to the hospital as it is expressed. After the baby arrives home, he can learn to nurse on your breasts.

### 24. Do I Need To Stop Nursing When My Baby Begins Teething?

No. Most babies never think about biting the breast that feeds them. Others must be taught—by taking them off the breast immediately, with an emphatic "No!"; then continue nursing. It also helps to give them other things to gnaw on.

### 25. Can Mothers With A Breast Infection Continue To Nurse?

Yes. Studies have shown that women who did not stop nursing when they had breast abcesses had much shorter illnesses and were much less likely to need surgery. Continued nursing from the affected breast has no adverse effect on the infant.

### 26. Will Birth Control Pills Affect My Milk Supply?

Yes. Studies show that the pills directly suppress lactation. The doctor will usually suggest that you do not nurse, if you take the pill. However, some women have been successful if they have a good milk supply and if the baby is well adjusted to the mother's milk before she starts taking the pill.

### 27. Does Breast Feeding Act As A Means Of Contraception?

Yes, usually. However, some women can become pregnant while nursing. This is unusual before the first menstrual period, if a woman is nursing completely. Complete breast feeding delays the resumption of the menstrual cycle.

### 28. Will I Be Able To Nurse Even Though I Have Had Silicone (Envelopes) Enlargement Of My Breasts?

These envelopes are inserted underneath the breast tissue and should not interfere with nursing.

192

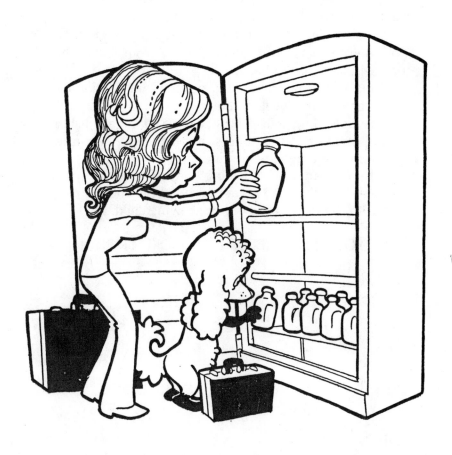

*If I Nurse—Can I Be Away From My Baby For A Few Hours Or Days?*

## SOME TIPS ABOUT NURSING

Some women have trouble with tender, sore, or cracked nipples, but these will heal if you persist.

The most important preparation is psychological. The most helpful person to talk with is a woman who has successfully nursed a baby.

Breast feeding can make a positive contribution to a child's emotional development.

Breast feeding in itself is not a prophylactic against the development of mental illness, but it produces optimum conditions for a healthy attitude.

The woman who is willing to give herself in breast feeding is on the road to motherhood—to the giving of herself to the total needs of her growing child.

## YOUR BABY NEEDS A "BOSOM" FRIEND!

# 26 | *Come As You Are—*
# *The Baby That Is*

The baby is going to seek its own most comfortable position regardless of whether this makes for a more difficult trip through the birth canal. About one in 30 will come as a breech—either feet or buttocks first.

A few will come out head first but looking upward (sunnyside up) instead of looking down. A rare few come in a position that makes delivery by way of the vagina impossible. However, your doctor can recognize and handle these variations.

**1.** *Can't A Breech Baby Be Turned So That It Comes Naturally?*

In a small percentage of cases it can be turned, but more often than not it returns to the breech position.

**2.** *Is It More Difficult To Have A Baby In The Breech Position?*

Yes, usually. However, with modern pain-relievers,

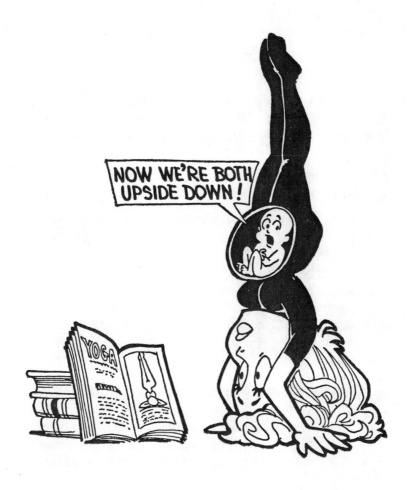

*Come As You Are—The Baby That Is*

nerve blocks and the other anesthesia, most women find little if any difference. It often means that a woman must work harder in order to get the baby down far enough in the birth canal for the doctor to deliver the baby.

### 3. Is It More Dangerous For A Woman To Have A Breech Baby?

The risk to the mother is very little if any greater than for other positions of the baby. However, the risk for the baby is somewhat greater with a mortality rate of 4 to 6%.

### 4. Why Not Have All Breech Babies By Cesarean Operation To Avoid That Risk?

Because the risk to the mother is greater in cesarean and many breech babies can be delivered quite easily through the vagina. The doctor's task is to decide which babies will be delivered easily and safely as breech babies and which require cesarean operation.

### 5. Are There Any Special Precautions I Should Take If The Doctor Finds That I Have A Breech Baby To Be Delivered?

You should report to your doctor immediately if your bag of water breaks. Since there is some increased risk of prolapse of the baby's cord (coming ahead of the baby so that its circulation could be pinched off), he will want to check you as soon as possible if your water breaks before you go into labor.

### 6. What Causes A Baby To Come In A Breech Position?

Sometimes a large baby's head in a small pelvis cannot descend through the birth canal. Because the baby's head doesn't enter the pelvis, the baby turns and allows the breech to descend into the pelvis first.

198

Other women simply have a pelvis that accommodates a breech position better than a head-first position. for this reason some women tend to have all of their babies in a breech position.

### 7. Does This Mean That I Will Have My Next Baby As A Breech Also?

If you have had a breech baby there is about one chance in five that your next baby will also be a breech.

### 8. Is There A Great Chance Of Injury To My Baby If It Is Delivered By Breech?

There is a greater chance for injury, but only if there is difficulty in delivery. Your doctor will decide if complications are likely. If there is any question in his mind he will perform a cesarean operation. Doctors usually lean very heavily toward a cesarean rather than take chances with you or your baby.

### 9. What Is A "Posterior" Position That I Have Heard So Much About?

Most babies are born head first and looking downward. However, about 10% are born looking upward, or at least they come into the birth canal in this position. Certain shapes of pelves favor this position.

By examination your doctor can tell if your baby is coming in this position. Many of these "posterior" babies turn over (rotate) spontaneously during labor and are delivered looking downward, which is an easier type of delivery.

Many of those that persist in the posterior position during labor can be turned by your doctor, either with his hand or, if this fails, with instruments. Certain "posterior" babies deliver very easily in this posterior position.

### 10. Why Is It Bad to Have The Baby In A Posterior Position?

The labor is often longer and may be more difficult and painful. The dimensions of the head in this position require more space to allow the head to pass through the pelvis and through the vagina.

For these reasons, a posterior may be a more difficult delivery, with a greater tendency to tears in the mother and injury to the baby. If possible a posterior position is usually converted by the doctor to an easier "anterior" position for delivery.

# 27 | *After My Baby, What?*

For the past several months, anticipation of having your baby has taken precedence over everything else. Would it be a boy or a girl, would it be normal, how would the delivery go? These questions crowded out other consideration—until now. Now that you have just had your baby—what next? What should you expect now and what about the future?

Every new mother faces a different challenge. Every doctor must decide what is best for his particular patient and her needs. Your problem may be different from all others. However, there are still many problems common to nearly all new mothers. Let's discuss a few of them.

## 1. *How Soon May I Be Up And About?*

This is the day of "early ambulation" in nearly every field of medicine. After a baby this means "as soon as possible," but may vary according to the type of labor and delivery you had and whether or not complications must be considered. Early ambulation may range from walking

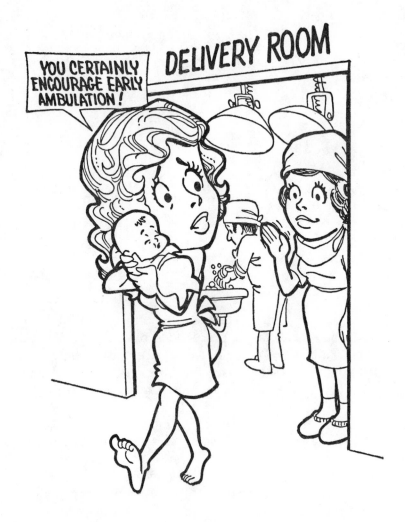

*How Soon May I Be Up And About?*

immediately and carrying your baby from the delivery room, in some instances, to remaining in bed for several days.

In general there are very few activities that you cannot undertake if you do them moderately. However, in YOUR particular case, your doctor must decide these things.

### 2. But Won't Everything Fall Out When I Am Up And Around?

No. This is a false idea, a remnant from the days when women remained in bed from two to four weeks after delivery. Nor will getting up cause you to bleed excessively—if you do it according to your doctor's direction and don't become overly tired.

### 3. How Soon Will I Begin To Look Normal Again?

At first your abdominal muscles will be flabby from being overstretched. However, with cautious exercising they slowly return to normal. At first you may wish to wear a supporting girdle to hold these muscles in. As you continue to exercise (types of exercises are discussed later) the muscles gradually regain their former tone and your figure will return to its former contours.

### 4. How Long Will It Take My Organs To Return To Normal After My Baby Is Born?

In general it takes about six weeks for the uterus to return to its normal size and for the muscles of the vagina to regain their normal tone. This process of returning to normal is called involution. When it is delayed for some reason it is called *sub*involution.

### 5. Is There Anything I Can Do To Help My Organs Return To Normal Faster?

Rest, modest exercise and a well-balanced diet aid this process. Nursing your baby also seems to speed up involution and makes it more complete.

### 6. How Long Will I Have This Vaginal Discharge?

Immediately after your baby is born the discharge consists of pure blood. Gradually this discharge becomes pinkish, then brownish and finally yellowish-white. After the first day or two the discharge becomes odorous, yellowish-pink and may persist for four to six weeks. During this time the discharge gradually becomes odorless and eventually becomes white in color. Sometimes the discharge disappears completely.

### 7. What About Douching During This Time?

During this time, if all else is normal, your doctor may allow you to douche with a medicinal solution to help diminish the odor and discomfort of the discharge. However, do not douche without permission from your doctor.

### 8. How Long Will I Have Afterpains?

Not all women have afterpains, but these cramplike pains are Nature's attempt to help the uterus contract in order to stop the bleeding. It is similar to clenching one's hand around a soft tube.

Within a day or two the bleeding is usually under sufficient control so that the cramps (so-called afterpains) stop. If you have afterpains with the first baby, it is very likely that you will have them with subsequent pregnancies. They sometimes continue for several days, especially when a mother nurses her baby.

204

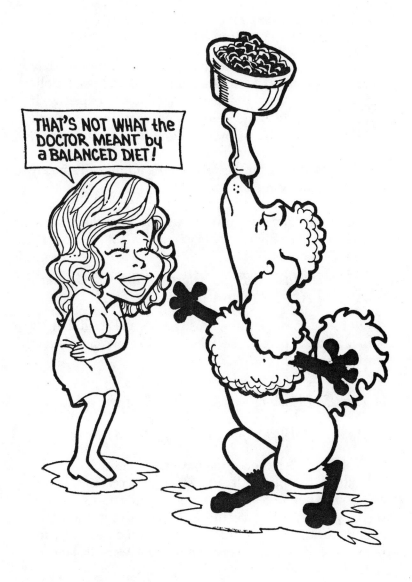

*Is There Anything I Can Do To Help My Organs Return To Normal Faster?*

9. *What Is This Lump I Feel In The Lower Part Of My Abdomen? It Is The Size Of A Large Grapefruit!*

That's a good description of the uterus immediately after having a baby, when the afterbirth and the amniotic fluid (water around the baby) have been expelled at delivery. Not only is the uterus large, reaching just about to the navel, but it also feels tender. It continues to decrease in size, rapidly at first then more slowly. Within ten or twelve days after the delivery the uterus can scarcely be felt in the abdomen.

Within six weeks time your uterus has usually returned to normal size, although it may never be as small as it was prior to the pregnancy.

10. *I Have Heard Of A Tipped Uterus. Will Being Up And Around After Having A Baby Cause This?*

No. As far as we know this is a normal condition for about 25 to 30 percent of women. It rarely causes any symptoms.

11. *How Can The Vagina Be Stretched Enough To Allow A Baby To Pass Through It And Then Return To Approximately Normal Size Again After Delivery?*

Not only does the vagina have great elasticity but it is also folded into pleats, like those of an accordion, which flatten out when necessary to accommodate the delivery of the baby. Pregnancy seems to provide any additional softening and elasticity of the vaginal tissue necessary for the occasion. The tissue tears when the baby is too large or the vagina is too inelastic.

12. *What About Stitches? Are They Really Necessary?*

The incision made by the doctor between the vagina

206

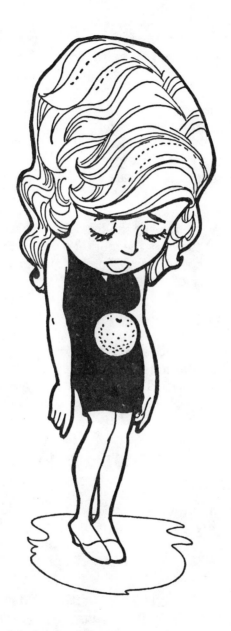

*What Is this Lump I Feel In The Lower Part Of My Abdomen? It Is The Size Of A Large Grapefruit!*

and the rectum at delivery is called an episiotomy. It is performed to protect your tissues from tearing or overstretching. Without an episiotomy the tissues underneath may be torn, even though there is no tear visible on the outside. Unless repaired, these torn tissues may not return to normal.

By cutting the tissues (performing an episiotomy) before delivery the baby can usually pass through the birth canal without overstretching or tearing the vagina. After delivery the cut muscles are stitched back to normal position.

In spite of the number of pregnancies, an episiotomy will usually help to protect the tissues and preserve better support for the "floor" of the mother's pelvis. By "opening the gate," so to speak, an episiotomy also makes possible an easier delivery of the baby.

### 13. How Many Stitches Did I Have?

Often the cut muscles in an episiotomy are stitched together with a continuous suture in several layers, one on top of the other, and in such a way that no stitches are visible on the outside. Therefore it is impossible for you to count the "number" of stitches.

### 14. Can Anything Be Done To Ease The Pain From Stitches?

Yes. Anesthetic ointments, sprays and lotions, as well as soaks, help to ease the pain from stitches. However, pain-relievers can be taken by mouth or even given hypodermically if there is undue discomfort.

### 15. I Am Worried About "That First Bowel Movement." Is It Going To Be Painful Because Of My Stitches?

Usually not. By alternating fecal softeners with large

208

amounts of water the bowel movement will pass easily and painlessly. However, be sure to drink plenty of liquids to give these fecal softeners something to work with. The softeners "draw" these liquids into the bowel, causing the fecal material to absorb them. In the process, the bowel movement swells up, becomes softened and easy to pass.

## 16. What Must I Avoid During The Next Few Weeks?

Women return to normal surprisingly fast. Check with your doctor because he may have special instructions. In general, however:
1. Avoid excessive fatigue.
2. Watch for pain and tenderness in:
    a. Abdomen—could mean infection in the pelvic organs.
    b. Breasts—could mean infection or abcess.
    c. Legs—could mean phlebitis (milk-leg).
3. If you begin to pass bright red blood, notify your doctor immediately!

## 17. How Can I Avoid After-Baby Blues?

These are common and many women have them to some extent. You must realize that there is a certain amount of normal "letdown" after being emotionally "charged" during your pregnancy.

However, avoid excessive fatigue and ask for help when you need it. There are also good medicines that doctors can use to prevent as well as to treat this condition in special instances.

## 18. How Can I Lose the Extra Pounds I Have Gained?

1. When nursing, remember that a mother needs only drink lots of fluids to make milk. She does not have to "eat for two."

2. When not nursing, here are a few rules to follow:
   a. Select low-calorie food and drinks whenever possible.
   b. Avoid between-meal snacks.
   c. Allow yourself one small helping. Sorry, no seconds.
   d. Avoid all fad and crash diets.
   e. Exercise regularly, preferably in the morning. This will keep you in better physical condition while you are dieting even though only a limited number of calories are consumed through exercise.
   f. Be realistic. Avoid discouragement. Set goals that can be achieved. Generally these are best regulated by the week rather than on a daily basis. A weight loss of 1 or 2 pounds per week is ideal, is not excessive and is better than a "crash" program.
   g. Lose weight without pills if you can do so. However, follow these rules if you need pills:
      1) Take them ONLY under a doctor's supervision. Your neighbor's pills may be perfect for her but poison for you.
      2) Pills should be taken only for a limited period of time, and a definite weight loss should be achieved. If continued indefinitely diet pills become ineffective and may be habit-forming.
      3) While taking pills, re-educate your eating habits to enable you to maintain your optimal weight once you have achieved it.
   h. If you diet for more than a month be sure to supplement your diet with vitamins.
   i. Weigh yourself at regular intervals. After all, the proof of weight loss is found in the pound—according to the scales.
   j. Calories do count, and they can add too—up to

210

pounds. (It takes 3,500 calories to "put on" or "take off" a single pound.)

### 19. How Soon May I Resume Sexual Relations?

Although there are exceptions, you should wait until after your checkup with your doctor. He can assure you that everything has returned to normal. You can also discuss contraceptives with him.

### 20. How Soon Is It Possible To Become Pregnant After Having A Baby?

Women have been known to ovulate (release an egg) in less than a month after delivery but usually it takes six weeks. To be safe and sure, it is better to use contraceptives every time.

If you will be using birth control pills you may begin taking them immediately after delivery, provided you are not going to nurse your baby. If you plan to nurse your baby, your doctor may want you to wait until after your lactation has been well established and your baby is getting a good supply of milk.

The pills can cause a decrease in your milk supply. A trace of the ingredients of the pill may also appear in the milk. It is not known what effect this might have on the infant.

Having a baby can be a great experience, especially if you know you can return to normal afterward.

### 21. About My Baby After It Is Born:
### A. Why Does The Baby Lose Weight At First?

Much of this is fluid in the tissues of the baby. Some doctors feel that the baby is "overhydrated"and loses some of the fluid as a normal course of events.

But you must remember that milk does not come

211

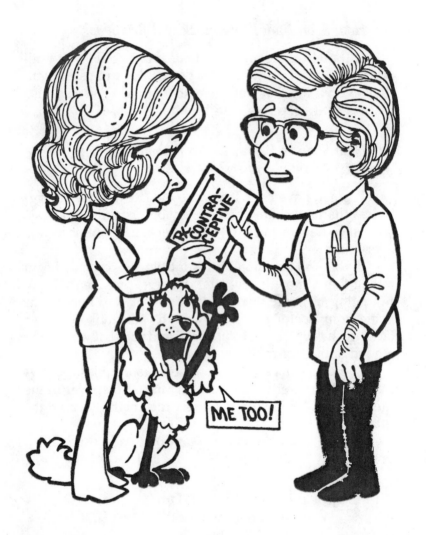

*How Soon May I Resume Sexual Relations?*

in for several days (two to four), in mothers who nurse their babies. In those mothers who do not nurse, the baby is not fed for 24 hours and even when fed, the baby takes very little formula for several days.

After the baby becomes used to eating and is somewhat stabilized, his weight soars rapidly. Birth weight is regained in about 10 days.

### B. Why Do They Put Drops In The Baby's Eyes?

This is required by law in some states to prevent any chance of gonorrhea from the mother being transferred to the baby's eyes. If untreated, gonorrhea can cause blindness in the baby.

### C. What About Belly Bands?

They are used only to appease the mother, but serve no purpose in the baby. They do not prevent hernia (rupture) of the navel in the baby.

### D. How Long Before The Cord Falls Off?

About three to five days. Ignore it unless the skin around it becomes reddened. Redness around the navel could indicate infection and should be reported to your doctor immediately.

### 22. How Soon Can I Use Internal Tampons?

This depends upon your individual case and your doctor. Let him decide when it is best for you to begin to use them.

# 28 | *Emergency Childbirth*

Modern transportation has brought nearly every woman within minutes of medical care. Do-it-yourself deliveries are becoming less common. However, campers and trailers have also enabled expectant mothers and their sports-minded husbands to venture far into our hills and deserts. Family boats take them up rivers and across lakes.

Actually, though, most women who start into labor can reach medical facilities, IF they don't wait too long to make up their minds to go. But we should know what to do in case of emergency.

Above all, remember that birth is a normal sequence to a very normal condition—pregnancy. If it is attended with difficulty, that difficulty will usually allow time to get to a hospital.

In the meantime, well—read the following pages.

## 1. Don't Panic!

The mother will reflect your condition, whether it be

one of composure or confusion and fear. If a baby is able to arrive before the mother can get to the hospital, it is nearly always a NORMAL birth. Talk in a calm, reassuring tone of voice.

### 2. *Try To Get The Woman To The Hospital If At All Possible.*

Many women who don't make it to the hospital, could have made it. Someone just thought they couldn't make it. If you can see that this is impossible, be sure to summon either the doctor or an ambulance. Even if late, the doctor can make sure everything is all right and the mother and baby are usually taken to the hospital even *after* delivery at home.

### 3. *How Do I Know If She Can't Make It To The Hospital?*

If the baby's head is beginning to protrude from the birth canal (vagina) then preparation should be made to deliver her where she is. Jostling of a speeding car or taxi at this point only complicates things.

### 4. *Make The Mother Comfortable.*

The most comfortable and safest position is lying down. She may feel as though she wants to empty her bladder or bowels, but this could be the uterus and baby bearing down. Have the mother use a bedpan or other basin rather than the toilet.

### 5. *Wash Your Hands Thoroughly.*

Soap and water are good preventives against infection. However, do not try to wash the mother. It is not necessary to touch her around the vaginal entrance.

215

*6. Protect The Bed, Floor, Or Even The Car Seat . . .If
There Is Time.*

Since there is usually a copious amount of fluid (water
and some blood) during a delivery, provide something to
absorb this. Newspapers, blankets, quilts, towels (paper
and cloth) can be used for this, but they should be covered
with a clean sheet or placed directly under the mother's
hips.

*7. Let The Baby Come Naturally.*

Nature will usually take care of this. The mother will
continue to bear down until the baby is expelled. Do not
pull, push, tug, or interfere. Just let her expel the baby onto
a clean towel or sheet.

If the mother happens to expel any bowel movement
along with the baby, this can be covered or removed so that
the baby avoids this contamination.

*8. Don't I Have To Help Deliver The Baby?*

Only rarely does it need help. In an emergency
situation it is usually better to let the mother expel the baby
by herself . . .without help!

*9. If The Baby Comes Out Encased In A Sac (Bag Of
Waters) That Is Still Intact, Break It!*

The sac is usually broken spontaneously in the process
of birth. If it is not, break it with your finger nail, a pin, the
tip of scissors or a knife. Then wipe the sac off the baby's
head. This allows the baby to breathe.

216

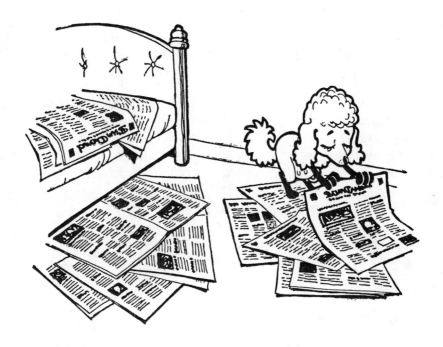

*Protect The Bed, Floor, Or Even The Car Seat. If There Is Time.*

10. *Wipe Off The Baby's Face, Including His Nose And Mouth, With A Clean Hankerchief, A Towel Or Even A Dishtowel.*

The purpose of this is to remove any thick mucus and allow the baby to breathe better. Don't use paper tissues that could get stuck in the nostrils or mouth.

11. *Place The Baby Alongside The Mother, In Close Contact With Her, If Possible.*

The best way to keep a baby warm is to place it in direct contact with the mother's body. If the cord is long enough, the baby can even lie on the mother's arm, next to her breast. If the cord is short, merely place the baby between the mother's legs... after you have removed or covered the secretions and fluids in the area.

12. *Do Not Stretch Or Pull On The Cord.*

Leave the cord slack, especially as long as it pulsates. This allows the blood to continue to flow *into* the baby. It is not necessary to cut the cord right away.

13. *Cover The Baby.*

This is for warmth. Use a warm blanket or a coat if nothing else is available. Do not cover the baby's head...leave room for it to breathe. Do not let the baby or the mother chill.

14. *What About The Cord?*

If the doctor will be able to arrive within an hour or so, leave the cord alone. The doctor will take care of this when he arrives

If he cannot be reached, tie the cord TIGHTLY in two places with a piece of string or strong twine. The closest tie

218

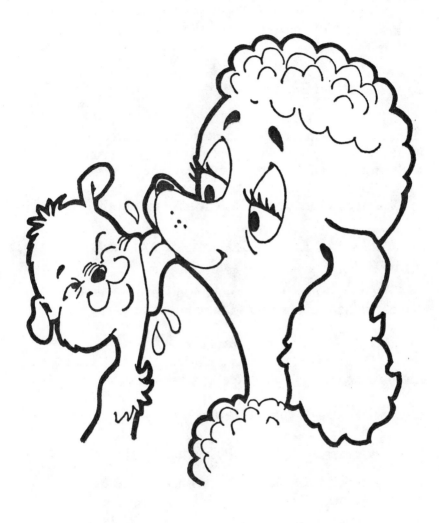

*Wipe Off The Baby's Face, Including His Nose And Mouth, With A Clean Handkerchief, A Towel Or Even A Dishtowel.*

219

to the baby should be about six inches from his navel.

Cut between the two ties with a clean pair of scissors or a knife. But remember that there is *no hurry* about cutting the cord.

## 15. *What About The Afterbirth?*

Usually the afterbirth is delivered by itself. When it comes, place it in a basin or a newspaper. Don't throw it away. Keep it for the doctor to examine when he comes. He will want to see if it is complete (that none of it is left in the mother).

Do not pull on the cord to deliver the afterbirth.

## 16. *Why Should The Baby Be Placed At the Mother's Breast?*

Even if the mother does not intend to nurse her baby, the baby should be placed at the mother's breast for two reasons:

a. This will keep the baby warm.

b. When the baby sucks at the nipple, it causes the uterus to contract, thus expelling the afterbirth. If the afterbirth has already been expelled, further sucking causes the uterus to contract to prevent undue bleeding.

## 17. *Is It Necessary To Massage The Mother's Uterus?*

It is usually wise to gently massage the uterus with a cupped hand after the afterbirth has been expelled. Sometimes the mother can do this better herself.

The gentle massage causes the uterus to contract and prevents excessive bleeding. After the uterus clamps down it will feel very firm and is usually about the size of a large grapefruit.

220

**18.** *Should Anything Else Be Done After The Birth Of The Baby And The Afterbirth?*

a. Clean the mother.

b. Make her comfortable and warm.

c. Do *not* clean the baby. It is better to leave the cheezy coating on the baby at this point.

d. Stay with the mother until the doctor comes.

e. If they are taken to the hospital, place a piece of adhesive tape on the baby's forehead with the mother's name written on it. This assures identification.

f. Relax and pat yourself on the back. All three of you made it!

# 29 | Miscellaneous Questions

### 1. What About Paint And Painting?

The bad reputation for paint in pregnancy originated with the fact that some women "drank" turpentine to provoke miscarriage. Naturally it caused a terrific intestinal upset and often resulted in miscarriage along with many other problems. In fact, if a person drank very much it even caused death.

However, there has been no proof that turpentine fumes from ordinary painting will cause miscarriage. If you do paint though, open your windows to avoid the nausea and headache that occasionally occur when inhaling such vapors. The newer waterbase paints have no odor or harmful vapors and require no precautions.

However, if you paint, be sure you don't fall off the ladder!

### 2. Is There Any Way To Avoid Stretch Marks?

Such marks result from rapid over-stretching of the

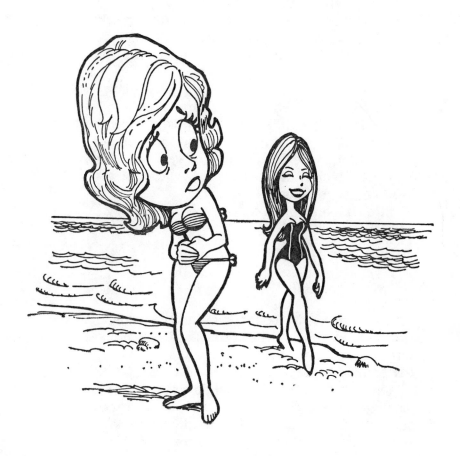

*Is There Any Way To Avoid Stretch Marks?*

skin. Normal skin contains elastic fibers that allow a certain amount of stretching. Some women have more elastic fibers than others.

But, when the skin is stretched beyond the ability of its elastic fibers to accommodate, the skin "breaks" and the reddened marks appear. These red marks gradually blanch out and become white in appearance, but they never disappear.

Fortunately they appear in areas that don't show (unless you are a go-go girl or a strip-teaser!)

Massaging, with or without cocoa butter or any other substance, will neither avoid nor remove such marks. Avoiding excessive weight gain will help, but often such marks depend upon the amount of elastic tissue you have inherited.

Stretch marks often cause intolerable itching.

**3.** *What Can I Do To Relieve Itching Skin, Particularly Around My Breasts, Abdomen And Hip Area—Especially Where Stretch Marks Are Located?*

There are many good lotions and even more theories about cures for this. First, make sure your soap is non-allergenic, and that you rinse your skin thoroughly after bathing or washing.

One of the best non-allergic preparations is rose water mixed with glycerine. Many pharmaceutical companies manufacture this lotion. If you do not wish to use this, choose a lotion or cream that agrees with you. For best results apply it to your damp skin.

**4.** *What About Dark Blotches Across My Cheeks And Forehead?*

This is often called the "mask of pregnancy" and also called liver spots by some, although the blotches

**224**

have nothing to do with the liver. They are common especially in brunettes, and there is no way to avoid them. Sunlight tends to make them more intense and noticeable.

Such marks gradually fade after the pregnancy, but have a tendency to persist in some individuals. Some of the blanching preparations sold on the market help to render the blotches less conspicuous.

### 5. Why Do I Have Such Large Veins In My Legs? Will These Disappear After My Pregnancy?

Due to loss of tone in the walls of the veins, they become stretched, allowing the blood to "puddle," especially in the legs. These veins become enlarged and engorged as they literally "sag" with blood.

Agreed that they also become unsightly. In fact, this may be the first thing women notice when they become pregnant.

Varicose veins are usually hereditary. Temporary relief may be found by elevating your legs as much as possible. Be sure your legs are higher than your pelvis.

If lying on a couch, drape your feet over the back of the couch. You can also place two pillows in the bed under your legs. Another method is to turn a kitchen chair upside down, place a pillow on the back of it, then lie down and place your legs over it.

If your doctor suggests elastic stockings, these should not be confused with support hose. Elastic stockings must be especially fitted to you and should be put on before getting out of bed. Support hose, by contrast, are sold in stores in small, medium and large sizes. Either or both may be effective.

Ordinarily these varicose veins disappear after a pregnancy. If they persist and are severe enough, they can be corrected by surgery. However, surgery on varicose veins is best deferred until after the pregnancy.

**225**

6.  *I Have Noticed That Many Pregnant Women have Swollen Legs And Ankles. Is This Normal For Pregnancy.*

Since nearly 80% of women have swelling we would have to say that this is at least average... and very common. Some of the swelling can be avoided by forcing fluids and avoiding EXCESS salt in the diet. However, a woman should not go on a salt-free diet while pregnant.

If swelling becomes so severe that the woman cannot tolerate it, the doctor may prescribe limited water pills. However, these must be carefully controlled and should never be taken without the doctor's permission... especially during pregnancy!

If the swelling is accompanied by elevated blood pressure or albumin in the urine it is more serious, since together, these are the signs of toxemia of pregnancy. See chapter on "Complications of Pregnancy" for more details on toxemia.

7.  *Why Does My Stomach Get So Hard? It Feels As Though I Might Be Going Into Labor, But Nothing Comes Of It.*

One of the common characteristics of the muscle in the walls of the uterus, is its ability to contract, rhythmically. This same rhythmic contraction in exaggerated form causes menstrual cramps as well as labor. Normally the uterus contracts rhythmically from the time of conception.

However, if the contractions become more severe, more frequent, and more uncomfortable, they are called "Braxton-Hicks contractions." They are usually harmless and disappear with rest or mild sedation. Only rarely do these contractions result in true labor and delivery.

226

### 8. Is There Anything I Do That Might "Mark" My Baby?

There is nothing we know of that will mark your baby. It is best to regard pregnancy as a normal state of being and continue to live just as though you were not pregnant.

### 9. Don't You Think That The Baby Is Affected By My Thoughts, Etc.?

If you are excited, afraid, etc., the baby might be more active within the uterus at that time, but there is no evidence that such an effect is lasting, as far as the baby is concerned.

### 10. Does It Matter In What Position I Stand, Sit, Or Lie Down As Far As My Baby Is Concerned?

No. Just as long as you are comfortable, the baby seems to adjust accordingly.

### 11. Is There Any Reason I Cannot Take A Tub Bath During Pregnancy?

It was thought at one time that tub baths might cause infection if water reached the vagina and cervix. This has now been disproved and pregnant women are allowed to shower or tub bathe as they please at any time during pregnancy until they go into labor.

In fact, a daily bath using a mild soap is advisable. However, you should be especially careful to avoid slipping or falling on the wet surface while getting in or out of the tub or shower. Use a rubber mat, or non-slip strips on the bottom of your tub or shower stall. Some

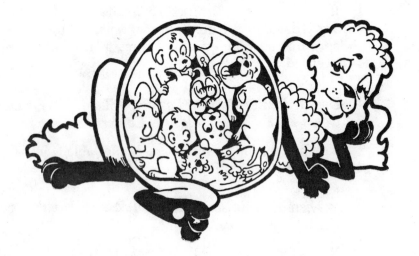

*Does It Matter In What Position I Stand, Sit, Or Lie Down As Far As My Baby Is Concerned?*

doctors prefer showers if the bag of water has broken, or if there is any bleeding.

## 12. Can A Baby Actually Have The Hiccups?

Yes, and some babies have them fairly often. The next time you feel a sudden activity in the uterus, take notice of such movements and you will see that they coincide with the usual rhythm of hiccups. There is no harm to hiccups, either to your baby or to you.

## 13. Is It Common To Have Increased Vaginal Discharge (With Itching) During Pregnancy?

. Yes. Because of the increased vascularity (greater blood supply) in these tissues during pregnancy, there is frequently a copious amount of vaginal discharge. Ordinarily this does not cause itching unless it becomes infected and the itching occurs when this vaginal discharge reaches the tissues outside the vagina.

Until you can tell your doctor about this discharge and itching so that he can treat your infection and relieve you of the irritation, you may try the following:
1. Keep the area clean and dry, but avoid too frequent washing, especially with a strong soap, since this washes away the normal protective oils in the skin.
2. Witch Hazel packs often stop burning and itching.
3. Ordinary petroleum jelly will offer some protection to skin from irritating discharge.

## 14. What Are Hemorrhoids? My Mother Said I'd Have Them.

Hemorrhoids are varicose veins of the rectum. Like other varicose veins, hemorrhoids are common during

**229**

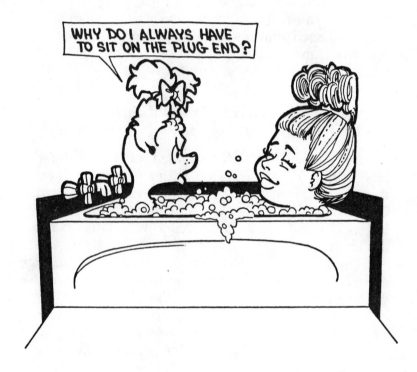

*Is There Any Reason I Cannot Take A Tub Bath During Pregnancy?*

pregnancy. This is not serious. A few suggestions may help to avoid them:

1. Develop a regular bowel habit—same time each day.
2. Drink plenty of liquids—preferably two quarts per day.
3. Avoid straining.
4. Use a stool softener in preference to a laxative.
5. Three tablespoons of honey a day prevents constipation in some women. This may be used in cooking or mixed with warm water or milk and taken at night
6. Elevate your feet (on foot stool, for instance) while sitting on the toilet.
7. Keep the area clean and dry. A cool Witch Hazel pack often gives temporary relief as suggested for vaginal discharge.
8. Anesthetic ointments, as prescribed by your doctor may relieve pain as well as itching.
9. Bleeding from the rectum should always be reported to your doctor.

### 15. Will I Have More problems With My Teeth During Pregnancy?

Not particularly, but you should remember to visit your dentist to have necessary dental work done. Good dental hygiene and a well balanced diet is your best assurance of a healthy mouth.

If you have done any vomiting be sure to rinse your mouth often and well, to avoid corrosive action of the stomach acids on the enamel of your teeth.

### 16. In Premature Babies, Does A Seven Month Baby Do Better Than An Eighth Month Baby?

No. This is strictly an old wives' tale. In general, the more mature the baby, the better its chances of survival.

**231**

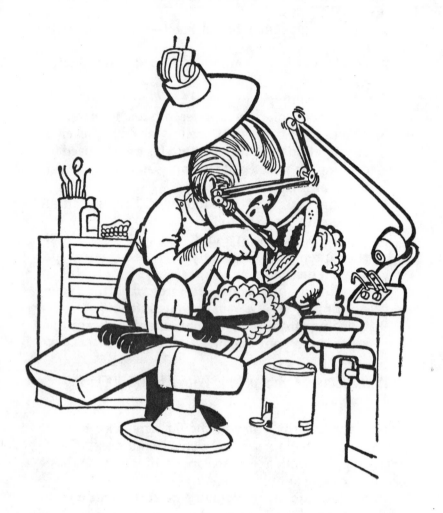

*Will I Have More Problems With My Teeth During Pregnancy?*

# 30 | *Contraception*

Aside from complete abstinence or surgical removal of the organs, there is NO absolutely 100% effective method of birth control or contraception. So-called birth-control pills more than any other, however, closely approximate this optimum. This, along with other methods and their effectiveness, will be discussed in this chapter.

## Safe Period

The method known as the "safe period" or the "rhythm method" is widely used, especially by certain religious groups who do not wish to use artificial methods of birth control. More accurate, however, would be the title, "relatively" safe period, for the average woman's cycle is unpredictable. Many women will occasionally be vulnerable or "unsafe," when according to the calendar, they should be safe from conception.

The rhythm method is based upon the assumption

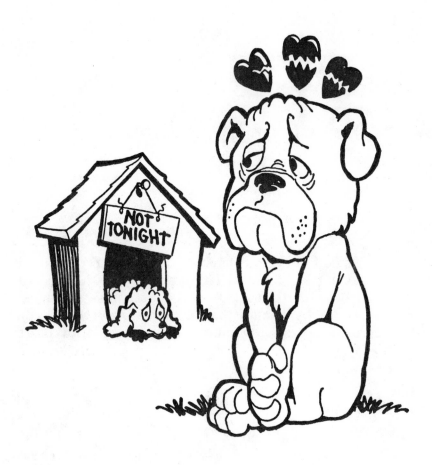

*Safe Period*

that the average woman "ovulates" or gives off an egg from her ovary every 28 days and that this ovulation occurs approximately 14 days before her next expected menstrual period is due to begin. Therefore, the "fertile" (or most "unsafe") time for a 28-day-cycle person is just 14 days before her next expected menstrual period, and in this case, 14 days AFTER her last menstrual period has begun.

On the other hand, if a woman has a 35-day cycle, her most fertile time would still be 14 days before her next expected menstrual period, but it now would be 21 days after the first day of her last menstrual period. The farther from this fertile time one departs, the "safer" the time becomes.

Hence, in a 28-day-cycle woman, the "safest time" would be just before and just after a menstrual period. Allowing three or four days on either side of the ovulation time as fertile, then any remaining days should be relatively safe.

One method of determining the safe period is to record one's temperature the first thing in the morning (preferably at the same time each day) and watch for the customary rise of four tenths to eight tenths of a degree at the fertile time. This same method may be used to determine the optimum time for conception as well as contraception.

## Condom Or Sheath Method

The male may use a condom, rubber sheath, or "prophylactic" as it is called, to contain the semen and sperm at intercourse to prevent conception. Such a method is effective and especially adapted to the couple in which the wife is unable or unwilling to use any contraception.

Precaution should be taken to check the sheath first to be sure there are no leaks and it should also be placed on the penis BEFORE coitus is begun. Many couples do not realize that the cause of their contraception failure is the fact that some sperm may be lurking in the male urethra and can effect conception WITHOUT ejaculation.

## Diaphragm With Jelly Method

A diaphragm used with jelly or cream is extremely effective and also is harmless as a method of contraception. The diaphragm must be fitted by a physician, but it is practically worthless unless combined with a jelly or contraceptive cream (other than petrolatum).

Generally speaking, a diaphragm cannot be fitted comfortably in a virgin because of the tight hymenal ring, but the bride can return to her doctor right after marriage for a fitting. At this time she should be instructed on the correct insertion of the device. Also she must know that the diaphragm should be left in place a minimum of eight to twelve hours after intercourse.

## Jelly Or Cream Alone

Spermicidal jellies and creams may be used alone without the diaphragm, but their effectiveness is decreased somewhat. Actually it is not so much the diaphragm that prevents the conception, but the spermicidal effect of the jelly or cream.

The diaphragm merely insures that the jelly or cream will be held in place. However, many women have used only these jellies and creams alone for many years, and swear by their effectiveness.

## Foams

With the advent of new packaging, it was only natural that jellies and creams would also be placed in containers with compressed air. Such a combination is the FOAM that is now so widely used. For the most part,

236

the effectiveness of foam approximates that of jelly or cream alone, but it may be more convenient to use. However, like the diaphragm, jelly, cream or condom, it must be applied BEFORE intercourse begins. Postcoital douching is best delayed until eight to twelve hours after intercourse.

## Suppositories

These are small pellets of low-melting-point preparations that can be inserted into the vagina prior to coitus. They promptly melt and provide protection equivalent in most cases to that of the jellies, creams and foams.

## Douches

The post-coital douche is as old as the contraceptive idea and has been effective for many women. However, it carries a fair risk of pregnancy and should not be relied upon as much as the aforementioned methods. Various preparations of all kinds have been used with testimonials for all. In general, the author cannot recommend these with great assurance.

## Coitus Interruptus

Coitus interruptus or withdrawal has been the commonest method of contraception known to man throughout the ages. In the average man who can judge the exact time of ejaculation, it has proved quite satisfactory and effective. The object is to withdraw the penis from the vagina just prior to ejaculation of the sperm, thus avoiding conception.

Although many husbands and wives find this method satisfactory, there are some disadvantages. First of all, it places a strain upon what otherwise should be an unstrained relationship. Both husband and wife may

**237**

worry about his withdrawing soon enough. Second, it prevents the husband from completing the act as he normally should. Just at the finest moment of their relationship, he must suddenly withdraw and "interrupt" the embrace.

There is considerable evidence to indicate a damaging psychological effect in some men because of coitus interruptus. In a sizeable number of husbands it is alleged to have caused impotence. It is simply not a healthy or normal way in which to end such an important process. Such an interruption may also prevent the wife from achieving her normal climax since withdrawal comes just as she is beginning or is in the middle of her orgasm.

Lastly, there are often sperm to be found in the normal male urethra that are extruded into the vagina BEFORE ejaculation of the male. These can effect conception, much to the consternation and puzzlement of husband and wife who have tried to be so careful.

## Intrauterine Devices

Intrauterine devices have been used for many, many years but have been frowned upon by most of the medical profession until the early 1960's. At this time new and safer materials and designs were introduced and the devices came into general favor.

These devices are produced in different sizes and with the exception of the steel ring, they are all made of plastic material impregnated with barium sulfate so they will show up on X-ray.

## Who Should Not Use An Intrauterine Device?

1. Those who have an active pelvic infection.
2. Those who have had no pregnancies may have difficulty wearing one because of pain, cramping

238

and the fact that the device is more likely to be expelled in these individuals.

3. Women who have distortion of the uterus by fibroid tumors may not have as much protection with an IUD.

## When Should The IUD Be Inserted?

Preferably two or three days after the end of a menstrual period. Following pregnancy it could be inserted during the first postpartum visit at either four or six weeks. Some physicians choose to insert them even earlier than this.

## What Complications Does One Have With The IUD?

Many women have none. However, here is a list of the commonest problems encountered with an IUD.

1. Bleeding. About 15% of the women have sufficient bleeding during the first year to require removal of the device. About 10% more have to be removed during the second year.

2. Expulsion. About 10% of the IUDs are expelled spontaneously during the first year but relatively few in subsequent years. However, a woman whose IUD has been expelled may be able to retain a second IUD that is inserted.

3. Some women have a considerable amount of vaginal discharge due to the IUD and occasionally this is sufficient to warrant removal of the device.

4. Pelvic infections are not common with the device but they do occur sometimes and may be treated with or without removing the device, depending upon the severity.

5. Extra-uterine pregnancy. Ectopic pregnancy may occur with an IUD because the device does not

**239**

offer protection against a pregnancy in the tube or the ovary. Although these are less common than without the device, they do still occur.

6. Perforation of the uterus. Rarely, about once in 2,500 insertions of the IUD, is a uterus perforated by the device. This can be serious and is usually recognized by the doctor, but pregnancy may occur if it is not recognized.

## Mechanism Of Action

No one is sure how the IUD prevents pregnancy, but most doctors feel that it hastens the passage of the egg through the tube and uterus and thereby decreases the chance of fertilization and implantation.

## How Safe Is The IUD?

Theoretically, the pill is supposed to be almost 100% effective, the IUD is 97.5% effective and the diaphragm and condom about 95% or more. For the woman whose body tolerates the IUD (i.e. does not bleed too heavily, have too much vaginal discharge with its use or expel it), it is the ideal contraceptive, for there is nothing the patient has to remember. Its presence is undetectable by either husband or wife.

If a woman becomes pregnant inspite of her IUD, she should report to her physician immediately to have the IUD removed. Otherwise she takes a great risk of infection.

## What You Should Know About "The Pill"

Several kinds of oral contraceptives are now available and your physician has prescribed for you the one he believes will best meet your individual needs. All types of oral contraceptives contain female sex hormones (estrogens and progestogens) and are designed to prevent the release of an egg from a woman's ovaries during the cycle in which the pills are taken. They are almost completely effective in preventing pregnancy.

"THE PILL" is the most effective of all contraceptives if you follow the directions for its use and are careful not to skip doses or take it irregularly.

Oral contraceptives, like all potent drugs, have some side effects. Fortunately, serious side effects are relatively rare. Periodic examinations, as recommended by your doctor, are essential to provide the early detection which may prevent serious complications. Report any special problems to your doctor.

## Common Reactions

A few women experience unpleasant side effects from the pill which are not dangerous and are not likely to damage their health. Some of these side effects are similar to symptoms women experience in early pregnancy and may be temporary.

Your breasts may feel tender, nausea and vomiting may occur, and you may gain or lose weight. A spotty darkening of the skin, particularly of the face, is possible and may persist. You may notice unexpected vaginal bleeding or changes in your menstrual period which should be reported to your physician.

Your physician may find that the levels of sugar and fatty substances in the blood are elevated. The long-term effect of these changes is under study.

Other reactions, although not proved to be caused by the pill, are occasionally reported: dizziness, changes in appetite, nervousness, some loss of scalp hair, increase in body hair and an increase or decrease in sex drive.

After a woman stops using the pill, there may be a delay before she is able to become pregnant. After childbirth there is a special need to consult your

**241**

physician before resuming use of the pill. This is especially true if you plan to nurse your baby because the drugs in the pill are known to appear in the milk, and the long-range effect on the infant is not known at this time. Furthermore, the pill may cause a decrease in your milk supply.

## About Blood Clots

Blood clots occasionally form in the blood vessels of the legs and pelvis of apparently healthy people and may threaten life if the clots break loose and then lodge in the lung, or if they form in other vital organs, such as the brain. It has been estimated that about one woman in 2,000 on the pill each year suffers a blood clotting disorder severe enough to require hospitalization. The estimated death rate from abnormal blood clotting in healthy women under 35 not taking the pill is 1 in 500,000; whereas for the same group taking the pill it is 1 in 66,000.

For healthy women over 35 not taking the pill, the rate is 1 in 200,000 compared to 1 in 25,000 for pill-users. Blood clots are about three times more likely to develop in women over the age of 34. For these reasons it is important that women who have had blood clots in the legs, lungs or brain not use oral contraceptives. Anyone using the pill who has severe leg or chest pains, coughs up blood, has difficulty in breathing, sudden severe headache or vomiting, dizziness or fainting, disturbances of vision or speech, weakness or numbness of an arm or leg should call her doctor immediately and stop taking the pill.

Women with high blood pressure should not take the pill.

## Other Considerations

If you miss one menstrual period and are following your dose schedule, you should continue taking the pill

242

as directed. If you miss a period, then you should stop taking the pill and see your doctor, even though you think you have followed the prescribed schedule.

There is no proof at the present time that oral contraceptives can cause cancer in humans. However, the possibility that they may continues to be studied, based on observations that large doses of female sex hormones have produced cancer in some experimental animals.

## Special Needs

If you have or have had a special health problem, such as migraine, mental depression, fibroids of the uterus, heart or kidney disease, asthma, high blood pressure, diabetes or epilepsy, inform your physician. He may wish to make sure that it is suitable for you to take the pill by doing special tests if necessary. All these conditions may be made worse by the use of oral contraceptives.

You should report to your doctor any unusual swelling, skin rash, yellowing of the skin or eyes, or severe depression.

There are some women, in addition to those with tendencies toward blood clotting disorders, who should not use oral contraceptives. These include women who have cancer of the breast or womb, serious liver conditions or undiagnosed vaginal bleeding when cancer has not been ruled out. It is comforting to know that, in such cases, your doctor can recommend other methods of birth control.

## Summary:

Oral contraceptives, when taken as directed, are drugs of extraordinary effectiveness. As with other medicine, side effects are possible. The most serious side effect is abnormal blood clotting. The fact is that serious problems are relatively rare, and the majority of women who would like to use the pill can do so safely and effectively.

See your physician regularly, ask him any questions you may have about the use of the pill, and report to him any special problems that may arise.

Perhaps no discovery in medicine of recent years has affected more people and their lives than the contraceptive (and controversial) pill. Even those who have not used it have had much to say about it. Many are the controversies that have arisen and these have not been confined merely to patients. Doctors, clergymen, lawmakers and even politicians have all entered into the foray. The final chapter is far from written, but we can discuss a few facets of this remarkable trouble-preventer or trouble-causer, depending upon our point of view.

The pill is effective as a contraceptive—almost 100% effective. Only rarely does a conception occur when it is used faithfully. It is convenient and requires only a good memory until the habit of pill-taking is established. Although it is usually well tolerated it does have a few disadvantages.

There are different brands of pills and dosage schedules; therefore, a woman should follow the directions outlined by her physician.

For the most part the pill prevents conception by preventing ovulation. It keeps a woman from giving off an egg, and without an egg "A hen cannot hatch a chick." However, forgetfulness in taking the daily pill may allow ovulation to take place and herein we have a built-in human hazard.

Ordinarily one day's dose can be missed without ovulation and consequent conception occurring. However, when a pill is forgotten, two pills should be consumed the following day. Failure to take several pills is usually followed by spotting or bleeding within two or three days. This is a built-in alarm to alert the woman to start taking her pills again and to use an additional method of protection for the next week.

The pill prevents ovulation, and thus prevents pregnancy. Women may experience side effects such as nausea, fatigue, weight gain, pigmentation of the skin, loss of libido, loss of pleasant disposition, to mention just a few. Occasionally some side effects are of a serious nature.

However, many women have NO untoward symptoms. And among those who do have such unpleasant symptoms a large percentage find that if they persist in taking the pills, they overcome all discomfort. Usually any discomfort is more than compensated for by the peace of mind women find in safety from conception.

However, there are important things you should know about the pill, and these may best be handled in question and answer form—

Q. Why are there so many different doses, strengths and combinations in various birth control pills?

A. Because not everyone reacts alike to a given birth control pill. For this reason, leave it up to your doctor to prescribe the proper birth control pill for you.

Q. If I forget a pill, will I get pregnant?

A. You certainly may be vulnerable, especially if you miss several pills early in any pill cycle. If you miss several pills in a row, you should expect to spot or even start to flow. What to do? Take two pills a day for two or three days and use an additional method of contraception for at least a week while you continue your pill schedule.

Q. What if I have spotting in spite of not missing a day with my pills?

A. This does not mean that you are or could become pregnant. Sometimes this happens, especially during the first month of pill-taking. What to do? Simply persist in taking your pills as directed.

If spotting persists for more than two months,

consult your doctor. He may change the dosage of your pill.

Q. What if I miss a menstrual period, even though I have not missed a day of pill-taking?

A. Occasionally this also happens to women who are not taking the pill. What to do? Continue to take your pills as scheduled to protect you from pregnancy. If you miss two menstrual periods, however, consult your doctor and he will tell you what to do.

Q. Should I take the pill at any special time of day?

A. It doesn't really matter when you take the pill, but take it at about the same time each day. Some women just starting to take the pill find they tolerate the pill better (less nausea) if it is taken with a meal, especially the evening dinner.

Q. Am I protected from pregnancy as soon as I begin taking the pill in the first cycle?

A. If you begin taking them on the 5th day of menstrual flow you will receive the full benefit of the medication for that month following. However, if in your first cycle of pills you begin after day 5 in order to start on a Sunday for instance, then you should use an additional method of contraception for one week. This extra protection would not be necessary after the first cycle of pill-taking.

Q. Is it possible that the pill can cause women who take it to become pregnant later in life, say at 65? That is, can taking the pill postpone the menopause?

A. This is not possible.

Q. Would there be any serious harm done if a child accidentally took a birth control pill?

A. No. However a child may get nauseous and vomit. If this happens check with your doctor.

Q. Do birth control pills cause twins, triplets, etc.?

A. No. You are thinking of fertility pills which are entirely different.

Q. Will the pills cause miscarriage if taken inadvertently by a pregnant woman?

A. No.

Q. How soon after my baby is born can I start taking the pill?

A. Since there are variable circumstances, each patient should follow the directions of her physician.

Q. Can I switch from one brand of birth control pills to another?

A. Yes. However, because of varying doses, you should do so only under your doctor's directions.

Q. How long may I continue to use the pill?

A. There is no limit. However, be sure to check with your physician each year or as often as he directs.

247

INDEX

C-8.758486821